# A Call to Action: Early Identification and Intervention for Autism in South Africa

Pauly

First Printing, 2024

# TABLE OF CONTENTS

# CHAPTER 1 INTRODUCTION AND LITERATURE REVIEW

## 1.1 Background

Autism Spectrum disorder (ASD) is a heterogenous condition characterized by persistent deficits in communication, social interactions and repetitive restricted patterns of behaviour that causes functional impairment (1). It greatly impacts on quality of life of the affected child, as well as that of their families. Signs of ASD usually develop in the first 2 years of life (2, 3), but most children are diagnosed from 3-4 years onwards. ASD has become a growing public health concern in recent years. In the United States of America (USA), documented prevalence in children increased from 1 in 150 in 2000 to 1 in 68 in 2017 (4-8). A systematic review of prevalence data in 2012 reported a global ASD prevalence of 0.6%, but noted limited data from Africa (5). Global developmental delay (GDD) is a neurodevelopmental disorder (NDD) category, where the child demonstrates significant delays in at least 2 domains of functioning, and some may manifest intellectual disability (ID) later in life. Estimate prevalence data in low income countries is lacking, but burden has been rising globally. In the sub-Saharan Africa, it was the leading NDD in 2014 (6, 7).

There is paucity of epidemiologic prevalence data of NDD in South Africa (SA). Despite the regularly held 'National Household Surveys' conducted by statistics SA, burden of disability in young children has never been captured at a population level. In one rural study done at Bushbuckridge, Northern Province, in 2002, they screened children aged 2 to 9 years for ID, and reported that 29.1/1000 had mild ID, while 6.4/1000 had severe ID (9). Another study done in rural SA in 2009 to determine the prevalence of NDD and behavioural problems in school children in grade R and 1 in Western Cape, authors reported that 21% had one or more possible developmental disability (10).

Children with ASD have complex care needs that require a range of health care services. Though not curative, early identification and intensive interventions can ameliorate some impairments. Behavioural intervention therapy directed at core ASD symptoms has the strongest evidence of effectiveness in managing ASD (11-13). Early intervention therapies including speech and language therapy, occupational therapy, physical therapy and psychologic interventions have shown proven benefit (14, 15). However, these interventions take time to show improvement and chronic management is required. Benefits of sensory integration therapy, and Complementary and Alternative medicine (CAM) approaches, and psycho-pharmacologic therapies remain controversial (16, 17). None the less, various studies have shown high use of psychotropics (18-21) and CAM therapies (22, 23) among children with ASD. A 2013 study in SA, observed high frequency of medication (24.6%) and CAM (40%) use in children with ASD (24). Children with GDD have similarly complex therapy needs spanning a long period.

Concurrent co-morbid conditions are common among children with NDD which further complicate their care needs (25). Medical conditions seen in ASD include gastrointestinal problems, seizures, sleep problems, allergies and recurrent infections which account for a large proportion of medical related visits (26-32). Co-occurring mental health problems reported include ID, anxiety, depression and attention deficit hyperactivity disorder (ADHD) (32-37). Behavioural problems in children with ASD frequently necessitate emergency care (26), and contribute to frequent health service usage (29, 35, 38). Co-morbidity patterns have varied across ethnic groups and geographic regions (27, 39). In a study done at a tertiary facility in SA in 2013 to characterize children with ASD, they reported a high prevalence of behavioural problems (89%), and most (72.4%) children in this cohort were non-verbal (40). Similarly, comorbidities have been described in children with GDD (25), but they often show fewer behavioural challenges. Problem behaviours may be misunderstood by staff not familiar with these conditions. Furthermore, these families often require other support services to assist them go through their challenges, and they still require primary health care visits for growth and developmental monitoring and vaccinations.

Studies in well-resourced countries have documented high service usage by children with NDD disorders compared to typically developing peers (41, 42). Children with ASD were reported have more challenges related to service usage, source of care, medical insurance and care coordination (43). Their hospital visits are costlier and these families are more likely to require government disability support than typically developing children (44, 45). Their care therefore poses a huge economic burden on insurance companies, society and to the government at large. The primary responsibility of accessing health services lies largely with families, who often report increased out of pocket costs in care, as well as reduced working hours and community participation. These factors contribute to higher stress levels, high frustration level, physical and mental health issues in these families compared to those of typically developing children (46-48).

These complexities raise the likelihood of unmet needs. Studies done in the USA have demonstrated substantially higher rates of unmet health needs in children with ASD compared to non-ASD children (49-51), and compared to children with other special health needs (CWSN) (52). Unmet needs reported included specialty services (49, 53), and therapy needs (53). The unmet needs increased as number of needed services increased, and especially in those with more severer limitations (51). There are limited services available in low resourced countries, hence greater care gaps are expected. In a study done in SA in 2009 to analyse unmet needs of disabled children, only 26% were receiving rehabilitative therapy and these were largely those with motor deficits (54). A study assessing services available for children with disability in Western Health Sub-district of Cape Town in 2014 reported that there were limited disability services, with few trained providers for the population needs and inadequate special education facilities (55).

Health service utilization (HSU) is a behavioural model that results from interrelationship of 3 variables; predisposing, enabling and need factors (56). From studies done in high income countries, need variables identified included disease severity, and comorbid conditions (51, 57, 58), predisposing factors included social-demographic and cultural factors (59, 60) while enabling factors included family income and possession of medical insurance (52). Health system factors also affect HSU. Among systemic factors reported in studies have included unmet expectations (38, 61, 62), limited knowledge by providers (53, 63), difficulties in navigating complex health systems (61, 64), and poor provider-carer communications (64, 65). The rising burden of these disorders are likely to impact on the provision and organization of services and costs of care (42, 44). Furthermore, poor service organization, inefficient systems, and bureaucratic systems are common system barriers.

There is a dearth of information on determinants of HSU by children with NDDs in resource limited countries. In the SA context, despite the rising recognition of these disorders in the community, the services available remain limited. Majority of affected households attend services in the public health system, where the initial evaluations and formulation of the management plan is done at a tertiary centre, then subsequently, core therapy and auxiliary services are accessed at community day hospitals (CDH), which are primary level facilities. Only a minority of cases attend care in the private sector, largely due to the cost restrictions. The rising service demand is likely to broaden the existing unmet needs, and increase disparities in access (54). There is currently limited information on how affected families juggle around these complexities to access care. This retrospective study reviewed HSU patterns of children with ASD and GDD accessing services at the Red Cross War Memorial Children's Hospital (RXH). We compared HSU between these two groups, and explored potential factors impacting on service usage. Findings will inform policy makers on appropriate structural organization for planning of future service delivery and resource allocation for more efficient services.

### 1.2 Rationale of study

In 2009, the estimated prevalence of NDD and behavioural problems among early school-age children in Western Cape was reported at about 21%, with ASD and GDD as the leading causes(10). Both children with ASD and GDD have complex service needs, covering core therapies, treatment for comorbid conditions, and other support services. These often require recurrent service use that spans long periods. These demand significant time investment and translates to substantial health care costs for affected families. Many households in low income countries have limited health financing, and even where services are state paid, overhead costs (such as transport), incurred by families pose significant barriers to care. Challenging behaviours are common among children with ASD, and often pose further challenges in their health encounters. Households with children with ASD therefore face more access barriers, compared to those with other NDD. Mostly, families are responsible for ensuring children attend services needed. However, when families feel overwhelmed, it may delay diagnosis, and lead to different care-seeking approaches, fragmented access, or discontinued care. Suboptimal care may result in poor outcomes, with lifelong dependency and disability lost years. Currently, all children with NDD receive similar health services. It remains unclear whether there is any meaningful difference in patterns of service use between households with children with ASD compared to those with GDD. This study sought to shed light on how these groups navigate their complex care needs. This will inform any additional supports needed to optimize access to care for these groups. There is scarcity of published studies in this area in SA, which underscores the importance of this study. This information is important for policy makers and health planners in planning for future health service delivery and refining pathways to care of these children and their caregivers.

### 1.3 Study goal

The goal of the study was to describe HSU patterns of pre-school children with primary diagnosis of ASD attending services at the RXH and compare with those with GDD (non- ASD), and to evaluate factors that influence these usage patterns.

### 1.4 Study Objectives

1. To compare frequency of HSU utilization of children with ASD and that of children with GDD at RXH.
2. To compare unmet health care needs for children with ASD and those of children with GDD at RXH.
3. To compare level of health service satisfaction by carers of children with ASD and those with GDD
4. To evaluate how socio-demographics, CAM use and family stress levels influence HSU patterns among children with ASD and those with GDD.

### 1.5 Hypotheses

*Hypothesis 1 (Objective 1)*

$H_0$: There is no meaningful difference in the frequency of HSU in children with ASD and those with GDD.

$H_a$: Children with ASD have higher HSU than those with GDD

*Hypothesis 2 (Objective 2)*

$H_0$: There is no difference in unmet health care needs for children with ASD and those with GDD

$H_a$: Children with ASD have higher unmet health service needs than those with GDD

*Hypothesis 3 (Objective 3)*

$H_0$: There is no difference in level of satisfaction with health services in children with ASD and those with GDD

$H_a$: Children with ASD have higher level of satisfaction with health services than those with GDD

*Hypothesis 4 (Objective 4)*

$H_0$: Families from low socioeconomic backgrounds (SEB) are more likely to have lower HSU than those from high SEB.

*Hypothesis 5 (Objective 4)*

$H_0$: Use of CAM by families is more likely to negatively affect HSU than those not using CAM.

*Hypothesis 6 (Objective 4)*

$H_0$: Families with high stress levels have higher HSU than those with less family stress levels.

### 1.6 Theoretical model

A modified version of Andersen's Behavioural Model of Health service (56) was used as the study frame work. This model proposes that health service use is a health behaviour that results from interaction of diverse variables that can be grouped into 3 categories; predisposing factors (static factors that describe the likelihood of an individual to seek care in a given situation), enabling factors (environment and resources available), and need variables (event or medical/ psychological conditions that might facilitate a greater need for services). Variables that were considered in these categories were as follows:

1. Predisposing factors: age, gender, race, family size, caregiver's marital status, education level, social supports, perspectives, previous health service experiences, level of satisfaction, use of medications and CAM therapies.
2. Enabling factors: Caregiver employment, family income, health financing, travel costs to the hospital, time taken to come to health facility, residence neighbourhood.
3. Need variables: Functional level or severity of illness, comorbid syndromic diagnosis, chronic medical and behavioural problems, emergency events, and family distress.

## 1.7 LITERATURE REVIEW

### 1.7.1 Introduction

This section examines existing literature on the subject under the following subheadings: health care needs of the children, effects of comorbidities on HSU, unmet needs in service use, HSU patterns among children with NDD, factors influencing HSU: sociodemographic factors, perspectives, stigma and preferences, family stress level and health system factors affecting service use, and provides a summary of gaps in existing knowledge.

### 1.7.2 Health care needs of children with ASD and GDD

Core symptoms of ASD include deficits in social skills and communication and repetitive restricted behaviours, attitudes, and interests. Intensive behavioural therapies have been shown to improve socialization and behavioural functioning (11-13). Early intervention therapy (EIT) covering occupational therapy, speech therapy, and physiotherapy have also shown significant benefit for better outcomes (14, 15). Educational and pharmacologic interventions targeting specific symptoms may be used in older children. However, none of these therapies are curative.

Services rendered often vary depending on the local resources. Clinical practice guidelines for ASD in the USA recommend provision of intensive intervention, with active management of the child at least 25 hours per week, 12 months per year (66, 67). Sustained and chronic management is required as interventions take time to show benefit (68). Children with ASD require more EIT, educational and behavioural services than children with other special needs (69, 70). Moreover, families may additionally require support services such as mental health care and family counselling. In many well-resourced countries, home health care services are available. However, in most resource-limited countries, a less rigorous approach is adopted, where the intensity and duration of therapy is unspecified.

Children with ASD suffer various comorbid medical conditions including gastrointestinal problems, seizures, sleep problems, allergies and recurrent infections, which account for a large proportion of medical related visits in this population (26-32). Most (87-97%), express diverse psychiatric comorbidities including; ID, ADHD, anxiety, behavioural and conduct problems and depression (29, 31, 35, 37). ADHD rates have ranged from 20-80% (29, 30, 32), while co-occurrence of ID has been reported in 50-80% (29, 36). Among teenagers with ASD, schizophrenia was reported in approximately 30% (71). In general, children with ASD express more challenging behaviours and emotional disturbances than children with other NDD (26, 35, 72). Gurney and colleagues (2006), analysing data from the National Survey of Children's Health, found that children with ASD had significantly higher prevalence of depression and anxiety (38.9% vs 4.9%), and behavioural or conduct problems (58.9% vs 5.2%) than children without ASD. They also reported that respiratory, food and skin allergies occurred more commonly in the ASD group, than other CWSN (25, 63). In another study by Horovitz and colleagues (2011), they observed that behaviour patterns varied between diverse ethnic groups in up to 5 of 10 domains tested (73). Mayes and colleagues (2011), examining predictor variables of ASD symptoms observed that behaviour and mood problems were significantly more common in children from lower socioeconomic backgrounds, controlling for gender and race. These groups also had more severer ASD symptomatology (74). Furthermore, Mandell and colleagues (2005), observed that African- American children and minority groups were more likely to exhibit aggressive behaviours than their white counterparts, but there were no differences observed in stereotypic and self-injurious behaviour (75).

Similar findings have been observed in low-resourced countries. Mpaka and colleagues (2016), looking at children attending neurodevelopmental outpatient clinics in the Congo reported high (93.2%) rates of comorbidity in children with ASD, but the significant comorbidity was with epilepsy (72.5%) and ID (75.8%), compared to children with other NDD ($p>0.001$). ADHD was reported in 14.5% and schizophrenia in 11%. The number of comorbidities per child ranged from 1-4, with more comorbidities reported in older children (39). Similarly, in a study by Springler and colleagues (2013) done in Western cape province in South Africa that examined children with pervasive developmental disorder, they a found high prevalence of behavioural problems (89%) and 72.4% were non-verbal (40). Belhadj and colleagues (2006) looking at a Tunisian population of children with ASD, reported comorbid ID in over 60% of cases studied, and 51.2% were non-verbal (76).

### 1.7.3 Effect of comorbidities and health service usage

Various studies have examined the effect of comorbidities on presentation and HSU. Problem behaviours in ASD may mask underlying medical conditions and delay diagnosis (77, 78).

Antshell and colleagues (2011), observed that comorbid psychiatric conditions were associated with latter ASD diagnosis and reduced symptom improvement (79). Comorbidities have also been associated with poorer prognosis (32). Most recommendations suggest that health care providers should pay attention and screen for comorbidities before starting any treatment for ASD (80).

Comorbidities often contribute to need for specialist and emergency visits. In a study done in the USA by Ahmedani and colleagues (2012), to characterize comorbid psychiatric conditions in children with ASD, they reported that 66.4% had a comorbid psychiatric condition. These tended to be those older, they suffered poorer outcomes, and were more vulnerable to recurrent service use than those without. This group was also more likely to be dissatisfied with services (38). Aggression has been shown to be one of the predictors of psychiatric hospitalization of children with ASD (81, 82). Children with more severer illness tend to have higher HSU (58, 83). Similar findings were observed by Zablotsky and colleagues (2015) in the USA, who reported that children with ASD and ID, especially those with co-morbid psychiatric conditions represented the most vulnerable population with recurrent service use and medication usage (84). Elsewhere, a Danish study comparing patterns of hospital contact of children by ASD versus non–ASD over a 10-year period, found that children with ASD had higher contact for diverse medical conditions than non-ASD children, both in periods before and after ASD diagnosis. They however, cautioned against using hospital data sources to correlate ASD with specific somatic diseases as this may be misleading given diverse criteria for entry to hospital care (85). From these studies, it appears that comorbid physical and mental conditions increase likelihood of service use in high income countries, but their impact has not been assessed in low income countries.

### 1.7.4 Unmet health service needs in NDD

From studies done in the USA, unmet needs in children with NDD have varied with type of services and child characteristics. Krauss and colleagues (2003) found that over one third of children with ASD reported experiencing problems accessing specialty care service, compared to just one fifth of children with ID and one fifth of children with other special care needs (49). Further, Chiri and colleagues (2012), assessed unmet needs and problems accessing core services (preventive, specialty care, therapy, and mental health) by children with ASD. They found that for this group, unmet needs ranged from 2.5% for preventive services, and up to 25% for mental health services. More unmet therapy and specialist needs were observed in children with ASD, than in those with other special health needs (CWSN) for all services (53). Benevide and colleagues (2016) examined population-based trend in unmet need for therapy service in children with ASD and CWSN and found ASD children to have 1.4 times higher risk of unmet needs (50). Similarly, Vohra and colleagues (2013) compared access to services, quality of care and family impact among children with ASD versus those with other NDD. They reported that children with ASD, were significantly more likely to report difficulty using services, lack of sources of care, inadequate insurance cover, lack of shared decision-making and care coordination and adverse family impact compared to children with NDD or ID alone (43). Warfield and colleagues (2006) in the USA examined service use by CWSN and reported that as the number of needed services increased, so did the number of unmet needs. This increased to 25% for children requiring 5 or more services. The authors also noted that mental health and home health services were the leading unmet needs (51). Common predictors for unmet needs for CWSN was low incomes and lack of insurance (62, 86). Other studies looking at all CWSN, reported that those with severer limitation of activities tended to have greater unmet needs than those with fewer limitations, and that they were also more likely to have delayed or forgone care entirely (51, 87).

Many low-resourced countries have limited services available for children with NDD. In SA, Grover and colleagues (1987) described services available for children with ID in Cape Town and demonstrated significant disparities between ethnic groups, and a serious under provision of services for the black African population (88). Subsequently, Redfern (2014) assessed disability prevalence in children accessing various services in Western Health Sub-district of Cape Town and sought to establish services available them. He reported that there were limited disability services, with few trained providers for the population needs and inadequate special education facilities (55). In study done by Saloogee and colleagues (2009) to analyse unmet needs of disabled children in peri-urban township setting in Gauteng, they reported that only 26% were receiving rehabilitative therapy. Those with motor impairments were more likely to receive therapy compared to those with intellectual impairment (44% vs. 8%, $p<0.0001$). In this study, only 26% of those that required assistive devices were receiving them (54). None of these studies looked at the ASD group specifically, yet they appear to be a particularly vulnerable group, given the above stated literature.

### 1.7.5 Patterns of health services utilization by children with NDD

Available literature on HSU by children with ASD originates largely from high-resourced countries (43, 60, 84, 89-94). Most analyses have focused on administrative database records, which may not capture family centred variables. These studies have focused on outpatient visits, emergency department visits and hospitalizations.

#### *1.7.5.1. Outpatient health service use patterns*

Gurney and colleagues (2006) undertook a large cross sectional survey of data from the National Survey of Children's Health 2003-2004, over a 12 month period, which revealed that children with ASD had a significantly ($p<0.001$) higher mean number of physicians visits for preventive care, non-emergency care, and emergency department (ED) visits than typically developing children (63). Liptack and colleagues (2006) also examined data from USA national samples and compared children with ASD and those without ASD, and found that children with ASD had greater utilization of services in terms of annual outpatient visits (41.5 vs 3.3), annual physician visits (8.0 vs 2.2) and number of medications prescribed annually (21.8 vs 2.1) (42). Similarly, when comparing health service utilization of children with and without ASD in the same health care plan, Croen and colleagues (2006) found that children with ASD had substantially higher annual mean number of total clinic (5.6 vs 2.8), paediatric (2.3 vs 1.6) and psychiatric (2.2 vs 0.3) outpatient visits compared to those without ASD (44). These findings were further echoed in surveys using the North Dakota Medicaid health claims from 1998 -2004 (95).

A study by Akins and colleagues (2014), compared utilization of conventional treatments in pre-schoolers with ASD and those with NDD. They reported that children with ASD received more hours of conventional services compared to those with other NDD (17.8 versus 11;$p<0.001$) (96). Cummings and colleagues (2016), looking at multiple health systems in the USA (2009 - 2010) found that children with ASD had greater health care use in many categories, but were less likely to receive important preventive services including influenza vaccination and other vaccinations compared to typically developing children (60). Nageserwan and colleagues (2011), analysing the 2005 National Survey of Children with special health care needs, reported that children with developmental disabilities had 2.3 odds of having difficulties using services, compared to 2.6 in those with mental disorders compared to those with physical disability (97). In a systematic review by Tregnago and colleagues (2012) to asses of disparities in health care of individuals with autism in the USA, they found that children with ASD utilize a greater number of health care services compared to children with other developmental disabilities, and had higher health costs (86). Kraus and colleagues (2003) examined access to specialist services by children with special care needs. They observed that over one third of children with ASD, compared to just one fifth of children with ID and one fifth of children with other special care needs reported experiencing problems accessing specialty medical care services (49).

Similarly, hospitalization rates have been found higher among children with ASD children. In the USA, Birenbaum and colleagues (1990), reported that 10% versus 3% of children with ASD were hospitalised during a year period, compared to all children. Elsewhere, in a population- based study done by Arim and colleagues (2017) using administrative data to compare HSU in children with and without NDD in Canada, they reported that those with NDD had three times more hospitalizations and two times more physician visits than those without. They also had higher use of psychostimulants and specialists visits (41). The three leading diagnoses in those with NDD were neurotic disorders, personality disorders, and other non-psychotic mental disorders (7.9%), acute respiratory infections (3.5%), and general symptoms (3.3%). Peacock and colleagues (2012) compared effects of comorbid medical conditions on health expenditures in ASD vs typically developing children and reported that children with ASD were estimated to have more than 2 times higher annual hospitalization costs and six times higher annual medication expenses than typically developing children. Medication costs were largely due to psychotropic medications (45). From this available literature, it appears that in some studies in the first world context, children with ASD attend more visits, but on the other hand there appears to be some aspects of care which are relatively neglected, including important routine health care visits such as for vaccinations. Most of these publications are based on studies from high income countries, but there is a significant gap in the understanding of how these issues play out in low resource settings.

*1.7.5.2 Emergency department visit patterns*

USA based studies comparing emergency department (ED) visits in ASD versus non-ASD children have documented higher usage by children with ASD (26, 27, 98). Reasons underpinning these emergencies have largely been routine childhood illnesses and accidents or injuries (99, 100). McDermont and colleagues (2008) compared the type and frequency of injuries presenting to ED by ASD versus typically developing children. The relative rate for ED visit for injury was 1.2 after controlling for age and gender. Treatment for poisoning and for self-inflicted injury were both 7.6 times as frequent children with ASD (99). Subsequently, Kalb and colleagues (2016) assessed causes of paediatric injuries presenting to ED and reported that the odds of an injury related visit was 54% greater among children with ASD than those with ID, but 48% less in those without ASD or ID. Main causes of ED visits among children with ASD was self-inflicted injuries or poisoning (100). Innauzzi and colleagues (2014) reviewed the 2010 National Emergency Database to identify medical problems presenting to ED by children with ASD by age group. They observed that psychiatric presentation was highest in the younger ages (12-15 years), while epilepsy was the highest presenting problem in those above 16 years (26). Similar observations were made by Kalb and colleagues (2012), who found that children with ASD were nine times more likely to present to the ED with a psychiatric crisis compared to those without ASD. Externalizing symptoms such as severe behaviours, including aggression and self-injurious behaviours were the leading causes of ED visits (34). Weiss and colleagues (2018) reported that immigrants had higher risk of psychiatric ED use, probably because of lack of awareness of mental health services and resources to effectively find accessible community support services for their child (101). Deavenport and colleagues (2015) assessed factors associated with ED utilization and urgency of visits, using data from various hospitals in the USA. The top reasons for ED visits by children with ASD was upper respiratory infections, and they had 0.26 times more annual ED visits, and were 2.6 times ($p$<0.001) more likely to have non-urgent visits ($p$<0.001), and their visits were less likely to result in hospitalizations compared to non-ASD children ($p$<0.001)(102). This available data clearly suggests increased ED use by ASD children than those non- ASD in well-resourced countries, but there is paucity of data on patterns of ED visits in children with NDD from low income countries.

### 1.7.6 Factors that influence health service use

#### *1.7.6.1 Sociodemographic factors and service use*

Various USA based studies have analysed the social determinants of HSU among children with ASD. Socially disadvantaged communities had lower access and uptake of services (59, 103), and their diagnosis occurred much latter (104). Thomas and colleagues (2007) looking at access to autism-related services by families, reported that access to care was limited for ethnic and minority families with low parental education (104). Liptack and colleagues (2008) reported that they utilized fewer of early intervention ASD specific services and had more difficulty accessing services (65). Irvin and colleagues (2012) found that those in higher socioeconomic status (SES) were associated with receiving more types of services such as "Applied behaviour analysis (ABA) - based services, and occupational therapy, than those from lower SES (105). Zukerman and colleagues (2016) observed that poor families were less likely to believe that they could change their child's condition. Parents of minority were more likely to believe that the condition was temporary, compared to white parents. Those with less education and of lower SES were more likely to think that their child's condition was a mystery (106).

Kogan and colleagues (2005) examined the impact of underinsurance on health care access among CWSN. They observed that underinsured children were disproportionately represented in low income families and were significantly more likely than fully insured children to have unmet health needs and difficulty in obtaining specialty referrals (52). In a systemic review of disparities in health care access among families with children with ASD by Tregnago and colleagues (2012), they reported that high costs of care and lack of medical insurance were shown to limit access (86). In study by Chiri and colleagues (2012) examining unmet needs and problems accessing core services among children with ASD, they noted that lack of health insurance was a barrier to access (53). In Nyugen and colleagues (2016) reported that having public insurance was associated with having <15hrs/week of individual services while mother having a bachelor's degree was associated with having <15hrs /week of classroom-based services (59). Similar findings were reported in study to asses role of parental education on service delivery and outcomes in children with ASD, where high level of parental education was associated with greater service adequacy and number of services received (107). Durkin and colleagues (2015), explored barriers to screening and diagnosis of ASD in low income settings and observed that there exists significant disparities in autism research, and children from low socioeconomic backgrounds were less likely to be diagnosed (108).

Age of child has been correlated with service use. Cidav and colleagues (2013), examined differences by age in service use and expenditures and reported that younger age groups utilized more of community-based services unlike older children who were reported as using more restrictive, institution- based care (103). While examining age-related trends in treatment use among children with ASD, Mire and colleagues (2015) observed higher early intervention service usage among the younger children. Most access to care for treatments peaked in the preschool years and visit frequency decreased with age, except access to care for the use of psychotropic medications (83). One study also noted a general decline in utilization of health services in youth with ASD as they transition to adult care with the exception of ED visits (109).

Ethnic differences have been observed in early identification of ASD in USA based studies. Mandel and colleagues (2005), observed that different cultures respond differently to similar impairments of ASD, including interpretation of symptoms, family decisions regarding interventions, and interactions between families and the health care system (75). Ancestral status and ethnicity have also been shown to predict use of specialized diagnostic procedures required by children with ASD (92). Examining impact of ASD on the family unit, Kogan and colleagues (2008) reported that compared to white children, non-Hispanic black children were more likely to report delayed or forgone care, have no usual source of care, no personal physician or nurse, have difficulty receiving care, or lack at least one component of family-centred care (62). Culture and race have been shown to influence psychiatric comorbid diagnoses among children with ASD (110, 111). On the contrary, the study by Nguyen and colleagues (2016) evaluating sociodemographic disparities in service use by children with ASD, observed that black American children entered the intervention earlier, compared to white children (2 vs 2,6 years, $p$=0.001), but observed decreased access to mental health services by non-white children (59). Ahmedani and colleagues (2012) looking at service access for children with ASD and psychiatric comorbidity did not also find race to be significant predictor of service access (38). Magana and colleagues (2012), reported greater disparities in care for ethnically diverse children with ASD, compared to children with other disabilities (112). Generally, these studies from high income countries reported varied conclusions on the effect of ethnicity or ancestry on service use in children with NDD, and it is likely that other factors are likely to confound it.

*1.7.6.2 Family perspectives, experiences and stigma and service use*

'The Health belief model' (113) and the 'Theory of planned behaviour' (114) define and categorize which factors may lead to service use. The later focuses on how attitudes influence social behaviours. Family decision making and choices around service utilization is a health behaviour. Understanding family perspectives in ASD care and subjective norms around care of ASD is an integral to understanding HSU. Cultural differences in health care seeking have been observed across different communities (115, 116). Parents' perceptions of illness plays a crucial role in determining treatment decisions (106, 117, 118). Care priorities and preferences differ by families based on their perception of severity (117), as well as other contextual or competing pressures.

Several mental disorders (119) and ASD (120) are frequently attributed to supernatural and traditional forces in Sub Saharan Africa and in Asia (121); these include lineage curses, enemies, an action of the devil and a punishment from God. To date, no single specific biologic or aetiology of ASD has been confirmed, though genetic variations are increasingly getting recognized as likely causes of the ASD behavioural phenotype. Caregivers may hold divergent beliefs and misconceptions about perceived causes and prognosis of developmental disorders in their children (121, 122). Parent perceptions on potential causes of NDDs (and ASD in particular) have evolved (106, 123, 124), as the scientific community hypothesizes about the pathophysiologic mechanisms underpinning ASD has changed in the last 50 years. However, there is less investigation on how these family perspectives affect ASD care. Al Abner and colleagues (2010) studied this link between parent causal perspectives and service use found that beliefs have a strong effect on treatment use. They found that theories about both external and hereditary causality were associated with use of nutrition supplements, especially special diets and nutrition supplements (117). In a systemic review by Carlon and colleagues (2013), they reported that many factors influence utilization of treatments, and suggested that future studies should asses relative weighing of these factors when making decisions (125). Zucherman and colleagues (2017) reported that higher parent-reported severity of illness was associated with higher likelihood of using therapy and attending specialist provider visits (58). In a study by Chadeiz and colleagues (2018), to correlate maternal belief on ASD aetiology and HSU, authors reported that belief in environmental causes was associated with receiving >20hr per week of ASD related therapy, whereas believe in environmental exposures, vaccines and medication as cause of ASD, was associated with preference for CAM use (118).

Families of children with ASD experience high stigma universally, covering high income countries (106, 126-128), especially among immigrant communities (129, 130), as well as low income nations (47, 122, 131). Families have reported experiencing either internal stigma (feelings of shame and the anticipation of prejudice that prevents people talking about their illness and looking for help), and enacted stigma (such as evasion and discrimination) (61). A study by Divan and colleagues (2012) in India reported that families would be ashamed if a family member was diagnosed with ASD (132). Similar findings were reported in studies from Africa. Ambikile and colleagues (2012) in Tanzania, reported that caregivers of children with ID and ASD experienced social exclusion and discrimination (47). Tilahum and colleagues (2016), in Ethiopia reported high rates of stigma among caregivers of ASD children; 43% worried about being treated differently, 45.1% felt ashamed about their child's condition, and 26.1% made effort to keep the child's condition secret. This did not depend on the child's diagnosis, gender, of caregiver education level (all $p>0.05$). Reported stigma was significantly higher in those who sought traditional help ($p>0.001$), provided supernatural explanations for their child's condition ($p=0.03$), and families who identified as being part of the orthodox Christian faith ($p=0.02$). The families also reported unmet needs in education provision (74.5%), health service provider (47.1%), financial support (30.4%) and developmental supports (27.5%) (122). This literature demonstrates that family perceptions of illness and stigma appear to determine their service use, but this did not been assessed locally.

*1.7.6.3 Family stress level and service use*

Families of children with NDD report increased out-of-pocket costs in care, reduced working hours and labour force and community participation (62). Families of children with ASD experience increased risk of stress, feeling of frustration and isolation and physical and mental health issues and decreased quality of life compared to those with other NDD (46, 48). Societal stigmatization, coupled with high care demands often lead to high stress levels (133). There are differences in treatment access and utilization with parent mental health in children with and without ASD (63, 134). The Tanzanian study by Ambikile and colleagues (2012), examined challenges of caring for children with mental disorders, and reported that psychologic and emotional challenges observed included being stressed by caring tasks, and having worries about the present and future lives of their children. They experienced sadness and inner pain or bitterness due to the disturbing behaviour of the children (47).

Parental mental health has been shown to impact on access to services for children with and without ASD (62, 63, 134). Individuals with ASD experience a high frequency of negative life events, trauma, and greater stress when compared to typically developing peers (135, 136). The stressors are in turn associated with decreased social functioning (135), and depression (137) which may lead to greater ED use. Thomas and colleagues (2007) looking at access to care for autism- related services reported higher rates of general service use rates among families with higher stress (104). Similar observations were made by Lunsky and colleagues (2012), in a prospective study in Canada, that that looked at predictors of ED visits in children with ASD, with and without ID. They reported that life events predicted ED visits in individuals with ID (138). Subsequently, Lunsky and colleagues (2017) also looked at predictors of ED use among adolescents with ASD observed that families who reported that their families were experiencing distress at baseline predicted higher ED attendance (139). This literature from high income countries indicates that among families with ASD, family stress level increases the likelihood of recurrent ED visits. There is need for better understanding of how this plays out in local settings.

*1.7.6.4 Medication, CAM use and service use*

The lack of specific standards of care for comorbidities in children with NDDs are subject to use of both conventional and CAM use (84, 140-142). Higher CAM use has been observed in children with ASD, in 28-95% cases (143-145). Croen and colleagues (2006) reported that children with ASD were nine times more likely to use psychotherapeutic medications and twice as likely to use gastrointestinal agents than children without ASD (44). Similarly, a longitudinal study in Korea to asses psychotropic use in ASD children aged 3-17 years found 30% usage (18). There is little evidence to support efficacy of use of these treatments for core symptoms of ASD (140, 146). Controlled studies have found these therapies to be ineffective (16, 144). Hanson and colleagues(2007) summarized the many reasons given to explain why parents appear to employ CAM more regularly for ASD: lack of efficacy of conventional treatments, poor access to standard rehabilitation programs, lack of agreement as to what treatments are best, better comfort provided by CAM professionals, empowerment of families, preference for less invasive and more 'natural' remedies and dissatisfaction with complimentary care (144). Most families adopt multiple treatment approaches and may discontinue treatment if they do not see perceived improvement (147). The lack of evidence on effectiveness, together with unclear biologic determinants of ASD leaves parents in dilemma (35, 141). Safety concerns exist for some of these therapies.

CAM use has been shown to affect conventional therapy uptake in the USA. In a study by Levy and colleagues (2010), families experiencing long diagnostic delays were more likely to use CAM like supplements and delay onset of conventional care. CAM use was higher when access to conventional care was limited (35). Zuckerman and colleagues (2017) reported higher CAM use in first time mothers who felt unsure of the aetiology of ASD, compared to mothers who cited specific reasons and in those with severer illness. They also observed higher CAM use in those with more severe illness (94). On the contrary, in the study by Akins and colleagues (2014), comparing utilization of conventional treatments and CAM in pre-schoolers with ASD and those with NDD, they found CAM use to be similar in both groups, with ASD at 39.6% versus 30% in NDD. Higher CAM was observed in those using the most intensive ASD-specific services, those with higher level of parental education and in those of non-Hispanic ethnicity (148). This literature therefore remains inconclusive on how CAM use impacts health service use. In SA, a study by Louw and colleagues (2013), reported high frequency of medication use (24.6%) and CAM use (40%) in children with ASD, but they did not explore how the use of CAM therapies affected service use.

*1.7.6.5 Health system factors and service use*

Caregivers of children with ASD have reported diverse challenges navigating health care services (61). These have ranged from long waiting times to evaluation, disinterest of clinician in parent's core concerns and short consultation times (38). Some have reported poor communication and over-helming environments (64). Others report failure of health services to meet their expectations and dissatisfaction with services received (38, 61). Health workers may either encourage or disenfranchise individuals from engaging in treatment, especially those who require care across multiple areas. Lack of confidence in competency of providers have led to patients preferring to visit ED instead of primary providers (63, 149). Vohra and colleagues (2014), looking at the 2009-2010 National Survey of Children with Special Health Care needs in the USA observed that caregivers of children with ASD were more likely to report difficulty in using services, lack of source of care, lack of shared decision making and care coordination compared to those with other developmental disabilities (150). In a study by Chiri and colleagues (2012) comparing unmet needs and problems in accessing core services in children with ASD and those with other special needs, they reported that families with children with ASD were more likely to report provider lack of skills to treat the child as a barrier to obtaining therapy and mental health services. They concluded that organizational features of managed care programs and provider characteristics pose a barrier to accessing care (53).

Parent -professional partnerships (PPP) can be defined as relationships between parents and professionals that are based on respect, trust, and equality (151). Parents with high quality partnerships are more likely to be satisfied with their current services and less likely to express high level of unmet service needs (151, 152). Families were more likely to delay or omit services if they perceived a lack of communication and partnership with the providers (38, 153). Families of children with ASD reported experiencing less collaboration, more disagreements and more dissatisfaction with services they received (64, 65), reflecting poor PPP with their service providers. In a study done in the USA, to asses role of parental education, empowerment and professional partnerships, and on service delivery outcomes in children with ASD, high PPP was associated with greater service adequacy and number of services received and explained >12.8% variance of service adequacy above and beyond the controls (107). Similar findings were reported by Parish and colleagues (2012), when looking at the effect of health care quality on service utilization in Latino families: collaboration, culture sensitivity, and time spent with the child were significant mediators of the relationship between ethnicity and health care utilization (154). Family choices and use of services can be related to health care access and quality (106).

A few studies have assessed health systems challenges in children with NDD in low income countries. In Nigeria, Bakare and colleagues (2009) reported low knowledge level among health workers on existing services and laws governing services for children with special needs (120). Subsequently, Bakare and colleagues (2009b) observed that diverse false perceptions were held by health workers on aetiology, treatability and preventability of childhood ASD (155). In Kenya, Gona and colleagues (2015) reported that among teachers, clinicians and social workers, supernatural causes, witchcraft and curses were considered as possible causes of ASD, and treatments ranged from traditional healing and spiritual healing to modern treatments (131). In study done in SA by Saloogee and colleagues (2007) to asses unmet health, welfare and educational needs of disabled children, lack of money, limited awareness about available services and bureaucratic obstacles were the main reasons offered by caregivers for not accessing care (54). Therefore, literature from the in high income countries suggests that households with children with ASD report worser patient experiences and low satisfaction in health care, which impacts subsequent decisions in care seeking. However, despite varied perceptions and knowledge level among health workers in low resourced countries, there is limited information on how this affects service use in children with NDD.

### 1.7.7 Summary of gaps in literature

Most literature on HSU in children with NDD originates from high income countries where health and support system are substantially better supported compared to low income counties. Individual, family, and contextual variables contribute to health service usage. The divergent clinical profiles and comorbidity patterns in these groups have been shown to impact HSU. Most literature describes increased HSU by children with ASD, compared to those with other NDD, but substantial disparities were observed among minority groups and socially disadvantaged communities. Family perspectives and stress level have also been shown to influence service use. Low income countries are facing a rising disease burden and service demands, but availability of services remains limited. Low level of knowledge, cultural barriers and stigma are still rampant among communities, as well as among service providers. High use of psychotropics medications and CAM therapies has been demonstrated widely. Very few studies have evaluated how these variables impact HSU among children with NDD in LMIC. Inadequate data makes much of the proposed conclusions and statements made here conjectural. There is need to understand how all these important variables affect service use in local settings.

# CHAPTER 2.0 METHODOLOGY

## 2.1 Study design

A retrospective cohort study was conducted. We enrolled pre-school children with a primary diagnosis of ASD and those with GDD (non-ASD) attending services at a tertiary hospital at a ratio of 1:1. At enrolment, the child's diagnosis was taken as what was documented in their medical record. HSU was determined by retrospectively reviewing their medical record visits in the preceding 1 year.

## 2.2 Settings

The study was done at the Red Cross War Memorial Children's Hospital (RXH), a leading tertiary public health facility in the Western Cape province of South Africa. The developmental service is a multidisciplinary service that manages children with diverse neurodevelopmental disorders and other multisystemic disorders with comorbid developmental disorders. The service operates about 60 clinics per month, covering neurodevelopmental and cerebral palsy clinics. The unit serves up to 4000 visits annually, of which 1500 are non-cerebral palsy NDDs, and a third of these have ASD. The service assists with establishing government guidelines aimed towards optimal care in a resource poor setting.

In addition, the hospital also runs a general paediatric emergency department service on 24-hour basis and offers primary care services. The hospital also offers rehabilitation services and various support services. The centre receives referrals from various community day hospitals (CDH), and private health facilities within their catchment area in the Western Cape province. Following the initial assessments, children are often sent back to the referring centre for their therapy needs. The system offers at least of one therapy session per child monthly, for each of the core services needed, as the routine standard of care.

## 2.3 Variables

### 2.3.1 The dependent variables

The dependent variable was annual frequency of HSU, covering outpatient visits for core therapy, specialists, emergencies, and primary care visits, and hospitalizations. The secondary dependent variable was unmet health care needs.

2.3.2 The independent variables

The independent variables included household characteristics; socio-demographic, economic, perspectives, level of satisfaction and family stress level and child factors including primary diagnosis, disease severity, comorbidities, medication use, and CAM use.

## 2.4 Study population

The study population were preschool children aged 3-8 years, residing in the Western Cape province, and within the RXH catchment area, and who were referred to the developmental service for assessment, and had been diagnosed with either ASD or GDD.

## 2.5 Study participants and sampling methods

2.5.1 Sample size determination.

A sample size of 240 was used. Sample size calculations was specific to each main outcome, with alpha=0.05 throughout, and equal numbers of children with GDD and ASD (1:1) in the sample. The primary outcomes for hypothesis testing were number of health care visits over preceding 12 months covering the overall annual visits and within the subgroups of core therapy, specialist visits, emergency visits, primary care visits and hospitalization

Sample size calculations were given for each category based on assumptions for mean (standard deviation) number of visits per annum. As data for expected number of visits overall and within subgroups is limited for this context, several assumptions were made and variations in power projected by differences in assumption. A sample size of 240, was calculated to provide 90% power to detect a mean difference of ≥ 5 overall visits comparing ASD to GDD, assuming a greater standard deviation (15).

2.5.2 Sampling methods.

Purposive sampling was done. We enrolled consecutive eligible children attending the developmental services who meet the inclusion criteria. Sampling continued till the desired sample size was attained.

*2.5.2.1 Inclusion criteria*

Preschool children aged 3-8 years attending the developmental services at the RXH, whose medical record indicated a primary diagnosis ASD (with or without other comorbid NDD, such as GDD/ID, ADHD, learning problems), and those with a diagnosis of GDD (non-ASD), whose parents/caregiver consented to participating in study. Families with more than one eligible child were interviewed only once.

*2.5.2.2 Exclusion criteria*

The study excluded children with missing medical records, those that had been hospitalised, those not accompanied by the primary caregiver, institutionalized children, those with visual or auditory impairments, Down syndrome, and those whose parents/caregiver declined to give consent to participate in study.

2.5.3 Sampling procedures

Parents and/or caregivers were made aware of the research through posters in the waiting area. We sampled cases from children attending their scheduled appointments at the clinic. The researcher was not involved in the patient care during enrolment days. The researcher reviewed the medical records of all booked children and identified those eligible. These were then flagged to the research assistants, by a sticker placed on the folder. After completing their consultation session with the primary doctor, the research assistants approached those eligible and explained to them about the research study and sought consent. Those fulfilling the inclusion criteria were then ushered to a private room, where they were interviewed by the researcher, and were assisted to complete the questionnaire. Those who declined participation were reassured that there would be no penalty for non-participation.

## 2.6 Data collection techniques

***Primary diagnosis***

Evaluation and diagnosis of all children referred to the clinic is routinely done by a developmental paediatrician, and their findings documented in the child's medical record. The DSM-V diagnostic criteria was used to establish the diagnosis of ASD. This was a clinical diagnosis based on the child fulfilling all three categories of deficits in communication, social interactions, restricted repetitive behaviours, attitudes, and interests and/or abnormal sensitivity to stimuli. Children with ASD who had other comorbid NDD such as GDD/ID or ADHD were included. The diagnosis of GDD was based on the child having delays of more than 6 months compared to their chronologic age, in at least 2 domains of functioning, namely cognitive, motor, fine motor, language and social skills, regardless of the underlying cause, but who had no signs of ASD.

***Other measures***

Individual data collection was captured using a data extraction template. This was facilitated through 2 separate processes; Information about the child's diagnosis, clinical profile, and treatments were extracted from the child's medical records at the RXH. Attendance dates were verified with the hospital appointment records. Visits done to CDH was extracted from the appointment cards of the respective facilities. Verification was done during the face-to-face interviews. A structured questionnaire (Appendix 1) administered to the caregivers sought the following information:

***i. Socio-demographic factors***

These included household characteristics covering age, gender, ancestry, residence, family income, family characteristics, language spoken, education level, occupation of primary carer, carer supports and child characteristics.

***ii. Clinical diagnoses and ongoing treatments***

*Diagnosis:* Child's primary diagnosis, age at first diagnosis, duration since diagnosis, disease severity and immunization status were obtained from the medical records, including the patient-held Road-To-Health Booklet.

*Co-morbidities:* Any underlying syndromic diagnosis, comorbid medical problems and psychiatric diagnoses occurring in last 1 year, were obtained from the medical record, and as per parental self-report. Psychiatric and behavioural comorbidities considered included ADHD, anxiety, depression, intellectual disability, conduct disorders, elopement, and self-injurious behaviours. Occurrence of any emergency events in the previous 1 year were also documented.

*Medications and CAM use:* Use of psychotropics or other CAM therapies was established from history and/or from medical records. These covered psychotropics, anticonvulsants, melatonin, homeopathic remedies, supplements, and special diets such as gluten free or casein free diets.

***iii. Family perceptions, distress, experiences, and satisfaction level assessments***

'The brief illness perception questionnaire' (brief IPQ), was used to asses caregiver perspectives (156). This tool has been validated for use in diverse chronic illnesses. It was adapted for our local settings. The tool identifies 8 dimensions within the cognitive representation of illness as follows; 1) Consequences describes the expected effects and outcome of the illness, 2) Timeline describes how long the patient believes the illness will last, 3) Personal control describes the extent to which patient believes that they have control over the illness, 4) Treatment control describes the extent to which patient believes that the treatment can control the illness, 5) Identity, describes how much the person experiences the symptoms of illness, 6) Concern describes how much the patient is concerned about illness, 7) Understanding describes how well the patient understands the illness, 8) Emotional response describes how much the illness affects them emotionally. The brief IPQ uses a single item scale approach to access perceptions in a continuous linear scale. Each dimension was scored on a scale of 0-4, with 0 as lowest and 4 as highest agreement, and the mean for each domain determined.

'The brief family distress scale for autistic children' (157) was used to assess family distress level. Caregivers were asked to rate their level of stress on a scale of 1-10, with 1 as lowest score and 10 as the highest level of stress.

'The brief questionnaire for assessing health care experiences (158) was used to asses caregiver experiences in health settings, with some local adaptations. Parents were required to rate their overall experiences during services accessed at the RXH and at the CDH on a Linkert scale of 0-4, where 0 = not satisfied, 1= somewhat dissatisfied, 2= somewhat satisfied, 3= satisfied, 4= very satisfied. The 5 subscales assessed included communication with therapist, communication with doctors, physical environment, management of disruptive behaviours at facility, and treatment communications by providers.

'The short- form patient satisfaction questionnaire' (PQS-18) (159) was used to assess client satisfaction with services. Parents were required to rate various services provided at the RXH and at the CDH, by stating how well their expectations were met, using a Likert scale of 1-5 (1= not satisfied, 2= unknown, 3= somewhat satisfied, 4= satisfied, 5= very satisfied), by responding to 18 questions covering 7 subscales; general satisfaction, technical quality, interpersonal manner, communication, financial status, time spent with doctor, accessibility and convenience, and overall satisfaction. The average of the scores for the 2 sites provided the final satisfaction rating.

***Outcome measures***

The primary outcome was the annual frequency of health service utilization, overall and within the sub-type of health care. Service areas covered included (1) core therapy visits, (2) specialist services, (3) emergency visits (4) primary care visits, and (5) hospital admissions attended in the previous 1 year.

*Core therapy visits:* Annual frequency of visits for physiotherapy, occupational therapy and speech and language therapy, was determined and corroborated by child's medical records. Annual attendance for ancillary support services such as social worker, counselling services, dietician, electrophysiology, and audiology services was determined.

*Specialist visits:* Visits to specialist clinics including developmental, neurology, psychiatry, genetics, allergy, gastroenterology, cardiac, surgical, dental, and other services in the previous year were documented.

*Emergency visits:* Frequency of visits to emergency department in previous year was documented. Parents were asked to state place where emergency services were sought, preferred point of services in emergencies, and whether child required admission.

*Primary care visits:* Families were asked to state if they attended any routine health supervision /vaccination clinics in the previous year and the type of services they had received. Verification was done by checking the Road-to-Health Booklet.

*Hospitalizations* – The number of in-patient admissions for more than 24 hours in preceding year at the RXH or any other hospital, was determined from the medical record, and by patient reports.

*Unmet needs* - These included services required but no appointment had been issued, or scheduled appointments that were missed for whatever reason, or therapy services missed, based on a minimum standard of once monthly schedules, but were not accessed.

## 2.7 Validity

All questionnaires used in the study including: the brief illness perception questionnaire, the brief family distress scale, the brief questionnaire for assessing health care experiences, the short-form patient satisfaction questionnaire have all been previously validated (156-159). 'The brief illness perception questionnaire' has been used in diverse chronic illnesses by Broadbent and colleagues (156). Specifically, use in autism was validated by Mire and colleagues (2018) in the USA (160). The patient satisfaction questionnaire has been shown to be adaptable, reliable, and validated tool for use in various settings by Thayaparan and colleagues (2013) in the United Kingdom (161). The brief questionnaire for assessing health care experiences in low income settings was validated by Webster and colleagues (2011) in Ethiopia (162).

The complete set of questionnaires were assembled into one unit and piloted on 5 mothers to identify potential ambiguities that needed to be addressed, and thereafter translation into isiXhosa and Afrikaans was done. Back-translated questionnaire were compared with the original questionnaire by an independent professional proficient in both languages.

## 2.8 Reliability

The final questionnaire was piloted on 10 participants to ascertain readability by layman level readers, clarity, and time of survey completion. Recruitment started by folder review by the researcher, to identify those eligible, by putting a sticker on their folders. Two research assistants who are qualified nurses assisted in the consenting of eligible respondents. Those caregivers that consented were requested to fill the questionnaires, and further interviewed by the researcher. For those with any missing data, the parent /caregiver was telephonically contacted to provide the information within 2 weeks of first interview.

## 2.9 Data Analysis

Exploratory analyses evaluated distributional properties of the main outcomes overall and within subgroups, including:

- (i) Count data for number of health care visits, overall and within subgroup of type of care
- (ii) Proportion of children with unmet health care needs
- (iii) Proportion of caregivers with high levels of satisfaction with health care

The main comparison groups were ASD vs GDD. Standard exploratory data techniques (EDT) were used to assess relationships between potential third variables and both the outcome and main exposure variables. Descriptive statistics were computed describing the sociodemographic characteristics, economic status, comorbid states, emergency conditions, functional level, medication use and parent perspectives, experiences, family distress level and service satisfaction level. In exploratory data analysis (EDA), health care visits were expressed as mean (standard deviation, SD), where normally distributed (difference in means compared with Student's t-test); or median (interquartile range, IQR) where skewed (equality of medians tested with Kruskal-Wallis). Categorical variables were compared with the $Chi^2$ statistic. Summary data has been presented in tables, pie charts and bar graphs. A modified version of Andersen's Behavioural Model of Health service (56) was used to group the variables into 3 categories; predisposing factors, enabling factors and need variables. The primary analysis used bivariable and multivariable linear regression to compare mean difference in visits between children with ASD and those with GDD (expressed as crude and adjusted beta coefficients representing mean difference in numbers of visits, with 95% confidence intervals). Multivariable models were used to adjust for confounders and test for effect modification of the main comparison (ASD vs GDD) by child sex, age group and maternal socio-economic status. Analyses were done in Stata version 14.0 (Stata Corps, College Station, TX); all p-values are two-sided.

## 2.10 Logistical and ethical considerations

Ethical approval for the study was obtained from the University of Cape Town, Faculty of Health Sciences Research Ethics Committee (HREC REF:397/2019) (Appendix 4) Approval was sought from RXH management where the study was conducted (Appendix 5). The study complied with the Declaration of Helsinki (2013). Written consent was sought from the parent/legal guardians to participate in study (Appendix 2). Strict confidentiality and privacy were observed during interview and data handling. Parents were free to decline participation without any repercussions. All children received the minimum recommended care during the study. Data was coded into a computer software program. Study findings will be published to benefit other children with similar circumstances.

# CHAPTER 3 RESULTS

# CHAPTER 3 RESULTS

## 3.1 Introduction

This section presents study findings under the following 6 subheadings: Sociodemographic characteristics, economic characteristics, child characteristics, family perceptions, family distress, experiences, and level of satisfaction and health service usage patterns. The effect of various family and child factors on HSU are then described.

## 3.2 Sociodemographic characteristics of study population

A total of 240 caregiver-child dyads were enrolled, 116 had ASD and 124 had GDD (Table 1). Caregiver's age ranged from 19- 58 years. Overall, the biologic mother was the primary caregiver for majority, (86%, 206/240) of the families. Regarding their marital status, 86/240 (36%) of the primary caregivers were single or separated from their spouses. While most (202/240, 84%) families interviewed were South African nationals, 16% (38/240) were foreign nationalities. The language spoken at home was predominantly English (91/240, 38%) or Afrikaans (90/240,37%). Most (204/240, 85%) of the primary caregivers had less than tertiary level of education. As pertains to availability of social support systems for these families, 79/240 (33%) reported having no other social supporter that could assist in bringing the child to the hospital in event of absence of the primary caregiver, and only 16% (38/240) having consistent support. Regarding any travel out of Western Cape province during the study period, majority (212/240, 88%) of the families reported having been away for a period of no more than 2 weeks in the preceding 1 year

Comparing the demographic characteristics of the two groups, they were found to be similar in most aspects, except for the availability of some social support, which was slightly higher in families with children with ASD, compared to those with GDD (86/116, 75% vs 74/124, 60%; $p$=0.04). The details of the sociodemographic characteristics are presented in Table 1.

**TABLE 1. Socio-demographic characteristics of study population by child primary diagnosis**

| | | Total (N=240) | ASD (n=116) | GDD (n=124) | P value |
|---|---|---|---|---|---|
| Age of primary carer (years) | < 25 | 15 (6%) | 9 (8%) | 6 (5%) | 0.77 |
| | 25 - 30 | 81 (34%) | 41 (35%) | 40 (32%) | |
| | 31 - 35 | 66 (28%) | 33 (28%) | 33 (27%) | |
| | 36 - 40 | 34 (14%) | 14 (12%) | 20 (16%) | |
| | 41 - 45 | 28 (12%) | 13 (11%) | 15 (12%) | |
| | > 45 | 16 (7%) | 6 (5%) | 10 (8%) | |
| Relationship to child | Biological mother | 206 (86%) | 101 (87%) | 105 (85%) | 0.66 |
| | Foster mother | 12 (5%) | 7 (6%) | 5 (4%) | |
| | Aunt | 7 (3%) | 3 (3%) | 4 (3%) | |
| | Grandmother | 14 (6%) | 5 (4%) | 9 (7%) | |
| | Other | 1 (<1%) | 0 | 1 (1%) | |
| Marital status | Married or cohabiting | 154 (64%) | 80 (69%) | 74 (60%) | 0.13 |
| | Single or separated | 86 (36%) | 36 (31%) | 50 (40%) | |
| Nationality | South African | 202 (84%) | 93 (80%) | 109 (88%) | 0.10 |
| | Other | 38(16%) | 23 (20%) | 15 (12%) | |
| Ancestry | White | 14(5.0%) | 7(6.0%) | 7(5.6%) | 0.55 |
| | Black | 134(55.8%) | 64(55.2%) | 70(56.5%) | |
| | Coloured | 89(37.1%) | 44(18.3%) | 45(36.3%) | |
| | Indian | 2(0.01%) | 0(0%) | 2(1.6%) | |
| | Other | 1(0.004) | 1(0.01%) | 0(0%) | |
| Home language | English | 91 (38%) | 49 (42%) | 42 (34%) | 0.49 |
| | Afrikaans | 90 (37%) | 43 (37%) | 47 (38%) | |
| | Xhosa | 42 (18%) | 16 (14%) | 26 (21%) | |
| | Mixed/other | 17 (6%) | 8 (7%) | 9 (7%) | |
| Level of education | Less than tertiary | 204 (85%) | 96 (83%) | 108 (87%) | 0.35 |
| | Tertiary | 36 (15%) | 20 (17%) | 16 (13%) | |
| Caregiver has a social supporter to accompany to hospital visits | None | 79 (33%) | 29 (25%) | 50 (40%) | 0.04 |
| | Sometimes | 122 (51%) | 64 (56%) | 58 (47%) | |
| | Always | 38 (16%) | 22 (19%) | 16 (13%) | |
| Time spent away from Cape Town in previous year | Never left Cape Town | 180 (75%) | 86 (74%) | 94 (76%) | 0.99 |
| | < 2 weeks away | 32 (13%) | 16 (14%) | 16 (13%) | |
| | 2-4 weeks away | 18 (8%) | 9 (8%) | 9 (7%) | |
| | > 4 weeks away | 10 (4%) | 5 (4%) | 5 (4%) | |

Numbers are n (column %) or median (interquartile range); p-values obtained from Chi2 test for categorical and Kruskal-Wallis test for equality of medians for continuous variables
All variables in this table represent data obtained from questionnaires completed by attending caregiver

### 3.3 Household economic characteristics of study population

Overall, families of children included in this study reported several economic challenges (Table 2). Overall, only 85(35%) of the 240 families had either the father or mother in formal employment, either on part-time or full-time engagement (Figure 1 and Table 2). Most families (210/240, 87%) reported a monthly income below R8000 South African rand (~ US$ 2020); 42% (100/240) lived in low-income neighbourhoods. The majority (170/240, 71%) of households used public transport to come to hospital, with some requiring the train service for part of the distances. Accordingly, the median travel time was 2 hours (IQR 2-2, indicating that at least 75% of the families travelled 2 hours), with most families requiring <R100 transport costs per hospital visit (91%, 219/240). A fifth of families (49/240, 20%) reported not receiving any governmental support for their child; 63% (151/240) were receiving the state paid childcare dependency grant, while 14% (34/240) were on social security for support (table 2).

Across measures, families of children with ASD tended to report more economically secure situations than families of children with GDD. This included higher employment rates (ASD vs GDD, 42% vs 29%; $p= 0.03$); and a higher likelihood of using their own car or a private (more expensive than public) taxi (ASD vs GDD: 38/116, 33% vs 23/124, 19%; p=0.008). Families of children with ASD were also marginally more likely to have an income of ≥R8000 than those of children with GDD (19/116,16% vs 11/124, 8%; $p=0.08$). Travel costs, time spent travelling and grant receipt did not differ by child primary diagnosis (table 2)

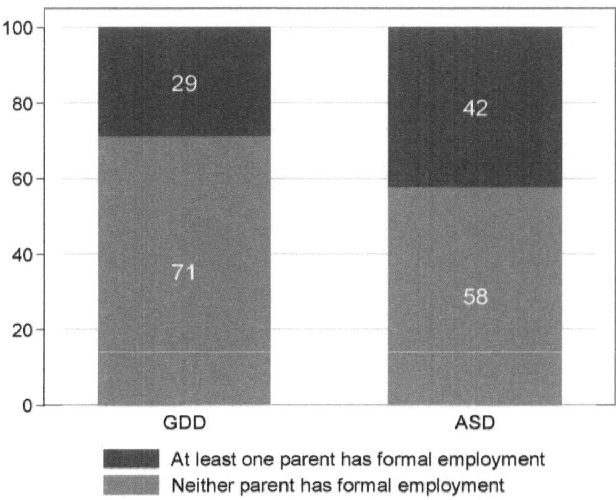


**Figure 1** **Parental formal employment (at least one parent vs neither parent) by primary diagnosis**

**TABLE 2. Household economic characteristics of study population by child primary diagnosis**

| | | Total (N=240) | ASD (n=116) | GDD (n=124) | P value |
|---|---|---|---|---|---|
| Parental employment | Mother and/or father have formal employment | 85 (35%) | 49 (42%) | 36 (29%) | 0.03 |
| | Neither mother nor father have formal employment | 155 (65%) | 67 (58%) | 88 (71%) | |
| Average family monthly income (Rand) | < R8000/month | 210 (87%) | 97 (84%) | 113 (91%) | 0.08 |
| | R8000/month or greater | 30 (13%) | 19 (16%) | 11 (9%) | |
| Type of neighbourhood | Low income | 100 (42%) | 40 (34%) | 60 (48%) | 0.08 |
| | Middle/high income | 140 (58%) | 76 (66%) | 64 (52%) | |
| Travel costs to and from hospital (Rand) | <R100 or unknown | 219 (91%) | 107 (92%) | 112 (90%) | 0.60 |
| | ≥R100 | 21 (9%) | 9 (8%) | 12 (10%) | |
| Means of transport | Walk | 9 (4%) | 5 (4%) | 4 (3%) | 0.008 |
| | Public | 170 (71%) | 73 (63%) | 97 (78%) | |
| | Own car | 49 (20%) | 34 (29%) | 15 (12%) | |
| | Private taxi | 12 (5%) | 4 (4%) | 8 (7%) | |
| Time spent to reach the hospital (Hours) | Mean time required to travel from home to hospital | 2 (2-2) | 2 (2-2) | 2 (2-2) | 0.58 |
| Mode of payment for healthcare costs | State paid | 191 (80%) | 90 (78%) | 101 (81%) | 0.83 |
| | Medical aid | 28 (12%) | 14 (12%) | 14 (11%) | |
| | Private insurance | 6 (2%) | 3 (3%) | 3 (2%) | |
| | other | 11 (5%) | 6 (5%) | 5 (4%) | |
| Does child receive any government support | None | 49 (20%) | 23 (20%) | 26 (21%) | 0.25 |
| | Social security | 33 (14%) | 15 (13%) | 18 (14%) | |
| | Childcare dependency | 151 (63%) | 72 (62%) | 79 (64%) | |
| | Other | 7 (3%) | 6 (5%) | 1 (1%) | |

Numbers are n (column %) or median (interquartile range); p-values obtained from Chi2 test for categorical and Kruskal-Wallis test for equality of medians for continuous variables

All variables in this table represent data obtained from questionnaires completed by attending caregiver

### 3.4 Child characteristics and diagnostic features

Overall, the children's age ranged from 3-8 years, with male: female ratio of 2:1 (Table 3). Majority, (157/240, 65%) were the only child in the household. Overall, most (145/240, 60%) had moderate disease severity. Parental concern was raised before the age of 3 years in 174/240, 72%), while in 66% (159/240) were first diagnosed before the age of 3 years. We reported syndromic diagnoses in 57/240 (24%), concurrent comorbid diagnoses in 65/240 (27%), and 82/240 (34%) were non-verbal. Most children (176/240;73%) were up to date on their immunizations.

As expected, there were some marked differences in clinical and diagnostic characteristics between children with ASD and children with GDD. Children with GDD were diagnosed at an earlier age than those with ASD ($p=0.0001$). Though the functional severity of the underlying condition was similar in both groups, higher co-occurring syndromic diagnoses were reported in those with GDD than ASD, (46/124, 37.1% versus 14/116, 9.5%); ($p=0.0001$), as well as more comorbid chronic medical conditions were reported in those with GDD than ASD (51/124, 41.0% vs 14/116, 12.1%); ($p=0.0001$) (Figure 2). More children with ASD had <10-word vocabulary at 62.9% (73/116), compared to 43.5% (58/124) with GDD ($p=0.01$). Though the use of prescription medications were similar in both groups, use of anticonvulsant medications was greater in those with GDD than ASD (16/124,13.0% vs 4/116, 3.0%); ($p=0.008$). However, use of CAM therapies was similar in both groups.

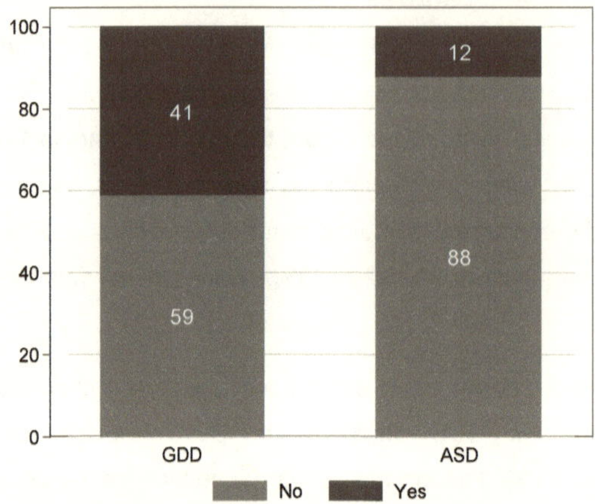


**Figure 2 Prevalence of concurrent chronic morbidity by primary diagnosis**

**TABLE 3. Child characteristics and diagnostic features by primary diagnosis**

| | | Total (N=240) | ASD (n=116) | GDD (n=124) | *P* value |
|---|---|---|---|---|---|
| Child age | ≥ 2 < 3 years | 28 (12%) | 12 (10%) | 16 (13%) | 0.41 |
| | ≥ 3 < 4 years | 29 (12%) | 11 (9%) | 18 (15%) | |
| | ≥ 4 < 5 years | 42 (17%) | 23 (20%) | 19 (15%) | |
| | ≥ 5 < 6 years | 71 (29%) | 40 (34%) | 31 (25%) | |
| | ≥ 6 < 7 years | 45 (19%) | 20 (17%) | 25 (20%) | |
| | ≥ 7 years | 25 (10%) | 10 (9%) | 15 (12%) | |
| Gender | Male | 164 (68%) | 87 (75%) | 77 (62%) | 0.03 |
| | Female | 76 (32%) | 29 (25%) | 47 (38%) | |
| Number of children in household | Only child | 157 (65%) | 71 (61%) | 86 (69%) | 0.19 |
| | Has siblings | 83 (35%) | 45 (39%) | 38 (31%) | |
| Severity of illness | *Level 1, Mild* | 38 (16%) | 17 (15%) | 21 (17%) | 0.58 |
| | *Level 2, Moderate* | 145 (60%) | 74 (64%) | 71 (57%) | |
| | *Level 3, Severe* | 57 (24%) | 25 (21%) | 32 (26%) | |
| Time of onset of parental concern | <3 years | 174 (72%) | 81 (70%) | 93 (75%) | 0.37 |
| | >3years | 66 (28%) | 35 (30%) | 31 (25%) | |
| Age at first diagnosis | < 1 year old | 46 (19%) | 8 (7%) | 38 (31%) | <0.0001 |
| | ≥ 1 ≤ 2 years old | 57 (24%) | 26 (22%) | 31 (25%) | |
| | > 2 ≤ 3 years old | 56 (23%) | 30 (26%) | 26 (21%) | |
| | > 3 ≤ 4 years old | 55 (23%) | 35 (30%) | 20 (16%) | |
| | > 4 ≤ 5 years old | 25 (10%) | 16 (14%) | 9 (7%) | |
| | > 5 years old | 1 (<1%) | 1 (1%) | 0 | |
| Congenital/ syndromic diagnosis | None | 183 (76%) | 105 (90%) | 78 (63%) | <0.0001 |
| | Genetic | 36 (15%) | 8 (7%) | 28 (23%) | |
| | Metabolic | 2 (1%) | 0 | 2 (2%) | |
| | Hormonal | 3 (1%) | 1 (1%) | 2 (2%) | |
| | Structural defects | 4 (2%) | 1 (1%) | 3 (2%) | |
| | Other | 12 (5%) | 1 (1%) | 11 (9%) | |
| Concurrent comorbidity | None | 175 (73%) | 102 (88%) | 73 (59%) | <0.0001 |
| | Asthma | 10 (4%) | 4 (3%) | 6 (5%) | |
| | HIV | 5 (2%) | 1 (1%) | 4 (3%) | |
| | Tuberculosis | 2 (1%) | 0 | 2 (2%) | |
| | Seizures | 18 (8%) | 3 (3%) | 15 (12%) | |
| | Other | 30 (12%) | 6 (5%) | 24 (19%) | |

**TABLE 3 (Continued)**

| | | Total (N=240) | ASD (n=116) | GDD (n=124) | *P* value |
|---|---|---|---|---|---|
| Verbal ability | Non-verbal | 82 (34%) | 45 (39%) | 37 (30%) | 0.01 |
| | < 10 words with meaning | 49 (20%) | 28 (24%) | 21 (17%) | |
| | 10-20 words with meaning, no phrases | 53 (22%) | 26 (22%) | 27 (22%) | |
| | > 20 to 30 words with meaning, 2-3 phrases | 29 (12%) | 6 (5%) | 23 (19%) | |
| | > 30 words with meaning, sentences | 27 (11%) | 11 (9%) | 16 (13%) | |
| Immunization status | Up to date | 176 (73%) | 82 (71%) | 94 (76%) | 0.42 |
| | Missed some | 39 (16%) | 18 (16%) | 21 (17%) | |
| | No recorded vaccinations | 12 (5%) | 8 (7%) | 5 (4%) | |
| | Unknown | 13 (5%) | 8 (7%) | 5 (4%) | |
| Prescribed medication | Any anti-epileptic agents (vs none) | 20 (8%) | 4 (3%) | 16 (13%) | 0.008 |
| | Any psychotropics (vs none) | 43 (18%) | 23 (20%) | 20 (16%) | 0.46 |
| | Any other prescribed medication (vs no other) | 35 (15%) | 12 (10%) | 23 (19%) | 0.07 |
| Reported CAM use | None | 173 (72%) | 83 (72%) | 90 (73%) | 0.73 |
| | Dairy restrictions | 16 (7%) | 9 (8%) | 7 (6%) | |
| | Other dietary restrictions | 33 (14%) | 14 (12%) | 19 (15%) | |
| | Supplements | 4 (2%) | 3 (3%) | 1 (1%) | |
| | Other | 14 (6%) | 7 (6%) | 7 (6%) | |

Numbers are n (column %) or median (interquartile range); p-values obtained from Chi2 test for categorical and Kruskal-Wallis test for equality of medians for continuous variables. All variables in this table represent data obtained from questionnaires completed by attending caregiver

## 3.5 Family perceptions, stress level, experiences, and level of satisfaction

'The brief illness perception questionnaire' (Brief IPQ) (156) rated 8 cognitive dimensions on a scale of 0-4. Overall, highest (163) rating was on "consequences" at 4, while the lowest rating was on "treatment control" and "understanding" dimensions, which were rated at 2. Ratings were similar in both ASD and GDD groups, except for the "understanding" dimension where the families of children with ASD rated it the lowest at 1 (Table 4). The components of the perception scores with medians and interquartile range are presented in Figure 2.

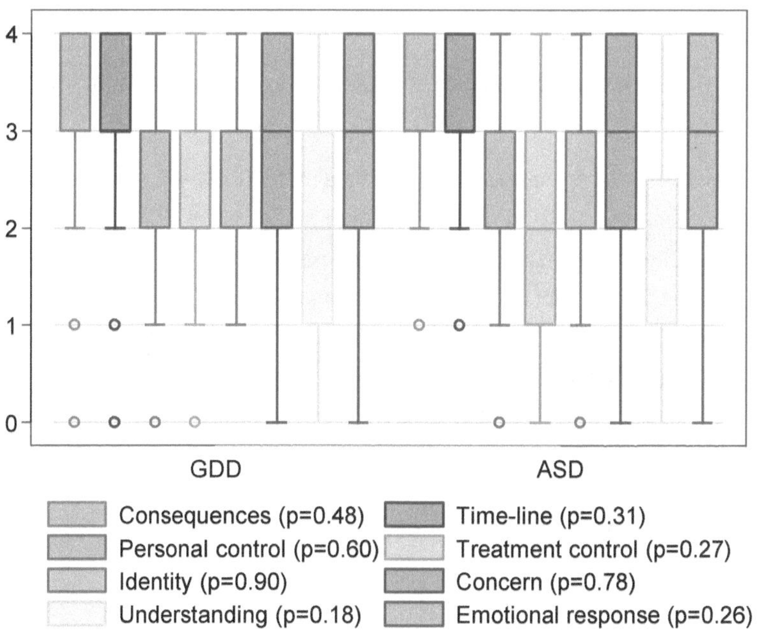


**Figure 3. Box-and-whiskers plots showing median (interquartile range) of scores for components of the Brief IPQ as completed by caregiver, by child primary diagnosis (ASD vs GDD)**

The mean score for this cohort on 'The brief family distress scale for autistic children' (157) was 3.3 out of 10 (SD 1.2). This score means that things are often stressful, but they were able to cope with problems as they arose. There was no difference in the mean ratings of stress level in both groups (Table 4). A few 3/116 (2.6%) families with ASD rated their stress level at 7, which meant that things were so bad for them and they would soon be in a crisis and they required referral to a family counsellor.

Parents rated 5 subscales on 'The brief questionnaire for assessing health care experiences scale' (158), using a Linkert scale of 0-4. Overall, the highest ratings were in communication with doctors and communication with therapists, both of which were rated at 4 out of 4, while the ratings for physical environment, management of disruptive behaviour and treatment communication of the home therapies were all 3 out of 4. There were no meaningful differences observed between families with children with ASD or those with GDD (Table 4).

Ratings on the 'Patient satisfaction questionnaire-18' (PSQ-18), were generally higher at RXH compared to CDH, but the average rating of the 2 sites was used in the analysis. Caregivers responded with mostly positive scores across domains (mean score above 3.5), except for financial status (mean score 3.4, SD 0.7), time spent with doctor (mean score 2.9, SD 0.7), and accessibility/ convenience (mean score 2.7, SD 0.1). High satisfaction (>80%), was reported in 8% (9/124) of families with children with GDD and 10% (12/116) of those with ASD. There were no differences by child primary diagnosis (Table 4).

**TABLE 4. Qualitative measures (caregiver perspectives, family stress, health care experiences and level of satisfaction) comparing families of children with primary diagnosis of autism spectrum disorder (ASD) to those of children with primary diagnosis of global developmental delay (GDD)**

| Scale name and items | Total (N=240) | GDD (N=124) | ASD (N=116) | Absolute difference (GDD- ASD) in means (95% CI) | *p*-value |
|---|---|---|---|---|---|
| ***Brief illness perspective questionnaire (B-IPQ)***[1] | | | | | |
| Consequences[2] | 4.0 (3.0; 4.0) | 4.0 (3.0; 4.0) | 4.0 (3.0; 4.0) | n/a | 0.48 |
| Timeline | 3.0 (3.0; 4.0) | 3.0 (3.0; 4.0) | 3.0 (3.0; 4.0) | n/a | 0.31 |
| Personal control | 3.0 (2.0; 3.0) | 3.0 (2.0; 3.0) | 3.0 (2.0; 3.0) | n/a | 0.60 |
| Treatment control | 2.0 (2.0; 3.0) | 2.0 (2.0; 3.0) | 2.0 (1.0; 3.0) | n/a | 0.27 |
| Identity | 3.0 (2.0; 3.0) | 3.0 (2.0; 3.0) | 3.0 (2.0; 3.0) | n/a | 0.90 |
| Concern | 3.0 (2.0; 4.0) | 3.0 (2.0; 4.0) | 3.0 (2.0; 4.0) | n/a | 0.78 |
| Understanding | 2.0 (1.0; 3.0) | 2.0 (1.0; 3.0) | 1.0 (1.0; 2.5) | n/a | 0.18 |
| Emotional response | 3.0 (2.0; 4.0) | 3.0 (2.0; 4.0) | 3.0 (2.0; 4.0) | n/a | 0.26 |
| ***Brief family distress scale***[3] | 3.3 (1.2) | 3.3 (1.2) | 3.3 (1.2) | 0.03 (-0.27; 0.34) | 0.80 |
| ***Experiences in Health Services***[4] | | | | | |
| Communication with therapist | 4.0 (3.0-4.0) | 4.0 (3.0-4.0) | 4.0 (3.0-4.0) | n/a | 0.73 |
| Communication with doctor | 4.0 (3.0-4.0) | 4.0 (3.0-4.0) | 4.0 (3.0-4.0) | n/a | 0.30 |
| Physical environment | 3.0 (3.0-4.0) | 3.0 (3.0-4.0) | 3.0 (3.0-4.0) | n/a | 0.77 |
| Management of disruptive behaviour | 3.0 (3.0-4.0) | 3.0 (3.0-4.0) | 3.0 (3.0-4.0) | n/a | 0.86 |
| Therapy communication | 3.0 (3.0-4.0) | 3.0 (3.0-4.0) | 3.0 (3.0-4.0) | n/a | 0.37 |
| ***Patient satisfaction questionnaire (PSQ-18)***[5] | | | | | |
| General satisfaction | 3.6 (0.6) | 3.6 (0.6) | 3.6 (0.6) | 0.0 (-0.2; 0.2) | 0.96 |
| Technical quality | 3.8 (0.6) | 3.8 (0.6) | 3.8 (0.6) | 0.0 (-0.2; 3.9) | 0.80 |
| Interpersonal manner | 3.7 (0.7) | 3.7 (0.7) | 3.6 (0.6) | 0.1 (-0.04; 0.3) | 0.13 |
| Communication | 4.1 (0.6) | 4.1 (0.6) | 4.1 (0.6) | 0.0 (-0.1; 0.2) | 0.77 |
| Financial status | 3.4 (0.7) | 3.3 (0.7) | 3.4 (0.8) | -0.1 (-0.3; 0.03) | 0.11 |
| Time spent with doctor | 2.9 (0.7) | 3.0 (0.7) | 2.9 (0.6) | 0.1 (-0.1; 0.2) | 0.53 |
| Accessibility and convenience | 2.7 (0.1) | 2.8 (0.8) | 2.7 (0.8) | 0.1 (-0.1; 0.3) | 0.41 |
| Satisfaction overall[6] | 23.9 (2.9) | 24.1 (3.0) | 23.8 (2.9) | 0.3 (-0.5; 1.0) | 0.51 |
| Proportion with high overall satisfaction (total score ≥ 28) | 21 (9%) | 9 (8%) | 12 (10%) | n/a | 0.60 |

Unless otherwise indicated, values are median (interquartile range) for variables with skewed distribution (p-values from Kruskal-Wallis test) or mean (standard deviation) for variables with normal distribution (presented in summary and with difference in means, p-values from t-test without ties)

[1] Scale ranges from 0 to 4, with 4 indicating strongest effects

[2] Missing data: n=1

[3] Scored from 1 to 7, with 1 "Everything is fine. Not in a crisis at all", and 7 "Things were so bad for them and they would soon be in a crisis"

[4] Scale ranges from 0 to 4, with 0 "Not satisfied" and 4 "Very satisfied; therefore, higher scores indicate better experiences with health care components

[5] Scale ranges from 1 to 5, with 1 "Strongly disagree" to 5 "Strongly agree"; therefore, higher satisfaction is associated with higher score; for analysis purposes, all non-integers rounded up

[6] Overall score from addition of 7 levels, therefore highest possible score is 35 and higher scores indicate greater overall satisfaction

[7] "High satisfaction" defined as having at least 28 overall score (28/35, 80%); that is, a minimum of 4 for all 7 levels of assessment; p-value obtained from Chi2 test

### 3.6 Health Service utilization patterns

The overall mean annual frequency of health care visits for this cohort was 12.4 (SD 5.7) visits per child per annum (Table 3). However, higher mean annual frequency of service use was observed for families with GDD (13.3 visits) compared those with ASD (11.5 visits), $p$=0.02. This primarily reflected differences in the number of specialist visits, with a higher annual mean frequency among children with GDD, 4.0 (2.0-5.5) compared to those with ASD 2.0 (2.0-3.0) ($p$<0.0001). The mean annual visits for other services were similar in both groups, including core therapy 6.0 (2.0-10.0), axillary services 0 (0-1.0), emergency visits 1.0 (1.0-2.0), and primary care visits 0 (0-1.0). Thirty-six (15.0%) children in this cohort did not attend any therapy in the preceding year, with similar proportions among those with GDD19/124(15.3%) and those with ASD 16/116(13.7%), ($p$=0.88). For those accessing therapy, frequency of visits ranged from 1-18 visits per child. Regarding access of auxiliary services, 37(29.8%) of households with children with GDD versus 27(23.3%) with children with ASD had accessed at least one of these services in previous year. Overall, 103/240 (42.9%) of the children in this cohort had attended at least 1 primary visit in the preceding year, comprising of 57(45.9%) with GDD versus 46(39.6%) with ASD. Emergency visits ranged from 0-10 visits per child per annum. While 23.4% (29/124) with GDD versus (22.6%) 28/124 with ASD had no emergency visits in previous year, 76.6% (95/124) of GDD versus 75.8% (88/116), with ASD had at least 1 emergency visit in the preceding year. The leading reasons for emergency visits for those with GDD were respiratory illness, unspecified fevers and seizures at 44/124(35.5%), 32/124(25.8%), 24/124(19.4%) respectively, whereas in the ASD group, was respiratory illness, unspecified fevers, and gastrointestinal problems at 47/116(40.5%), 25/116(21.5%) and 16/112(13.7%) respectively. Overall injuries or accidents accounted for 8.7% (21/240), while mental and behavioural problems accounted for 5.7% (15/240) of reported emergency visits in this cohort. Overall, 22.5% (54/240) of children had at least one hospitalization in the previous year. Hospitalization was more likely among children with GDD (38/124, 31%) than among those with ASD (16/116, 14%), $p$=0.02.

**TABLE 5. Health care utilization over previous year, by primary diagnosis: comparison of mean and median numbers of overall and specific health care visits comparing children with ASD to children with GDD**

| | Total (N=240) | Global developmental disorder (n=124) | Autism spectrum disorder (n=116) | Mean difference (95% CI) | *p*-value |
|---|---|---|---|---|---|
| Overall outpatient visits (sum of all attended visits)[1] | 12.4 (5.7) | 13.3 (6.0) | 11.5 (5.3) | 1.7 (0.3; 3.2) | 0.02 |
| Core therapy visits[2] | 6.0 (2.0-10.0) | 6.0 (2.0-9.0) | 6.0 (2.0-10.0) | - | 0.56 |
| Auxiliary service visits[3] | 0 (0-1.0) | 0 (0-1.0) | 0 (0-0) | - | 0.22 |
| Emergency service visits[4] | 1.0 (1.0-2.0) | 1.0 (1.0 -2.0) | 1.0 (0.5 -2.5) | - | 0.51 |
| Specialist visits[5] | 3.0 (2.0-4.5) | 4.0 (2.0 -5.5) | 2.0 (2.0 -3.0) | - | 0.0001 |
| Primary care visits[6] | 0 (0 -1.0) | 0 (0-1.0) | 0 (0 -1.0) | - | 0.26 |
| Hospitalizations[7] | 0 (0-0) | 0 (0-1) | 0 (0-0) | - | 0.02 |

Numbers are median (interquartile range) visits where variable distribution is skewed (p-value from Kruskal-Wallis equality of medians test), or mean (standard deviation) with p-values from T-test and presented with difference in means (95% confidence interval)

[1] Sum of core, auxiliary, emergency, specialist care and primary care visits

[2] Includes physiotherapy, occupational therapy, and speech/language therapy visits

[3] Includes appointments for audiology, social worker, family counsellor, electrophysiological monitoring and Dietician.

[4] Includes any health care visits for acute illness such as diarrhoea, pneumonia, seizures etc.

[5] Includes neurology, neuro-developmental, genetic, ophthalmology, gastroenterology, pulmonology allergy, cardiology, surgical (including ear, nose, and throat)

[6] Includes routine vaccination and clinic -level growth monitoring

[7] Includes admissions at any health facility for more than 24 hours.

### 3.7 Factors affecting Health Service utilization patterns

Factors associated with health service utilization (number of annual health visits) are shown overall, and within sub-groups of primary diagnosis (GDD and ASD), in table 6. Crude beta coefficients represent mean difference in average number of annual visits by comparison groups, obtained from linear regression; negative coefficients indicate lower annual HSU, while positive coefficients indicate higher annual HSU. Table 7 shows adjusted mean differences in average number of annual visits, obtained from multivariable linear regression.

Overall, children with ASD had 1.76 fewer annual visits compared to those with GDD (β -1.76, 95% CI -3.20 to -0.32; p=0.02). Unsurprisingly, factors known to be predictive of a diagnosis of GDD rather than ASD (and therefore reflecting the need factors associated with GDD) were also predictive of higher HSU in the overall cohort. In epidemiological terms, these factors emerged as confounders (and consequently associations were lessened or no longer present once analysis was stratified by primary diagnoses).These included being female (vs male, average 1.59 more annual visits, *p*=0.04), being younger at first diagnosis (<2 vs ≥ 2 years, 1.72 more annual visits, *p*= 0.02), and having a concurrent syndromic diagnosis (vs none, 2.19 more annual visits, *p*=0.01). Controlling for these factors in the multivariable analysis, parental employment emerged as the strongest residual predictive factor for increased HSU (β 1.49, 95% CI -0.02 to 3.00, *p*=0.05), table 7. Overall, other factors (associated with higher HSU) included marital status (married vs single/separated, β 1.61, 95% CI 0.11 to 3.11; *p*=0.04; a predisposing factor), and caregivers' higher belief that therapy was able to control the illness ("Treatment control", per unit increase in score: β 1.04, 95% CI 0.38 to 1.76, *p*=0.003). Figure 2 shows the median (IQR) annual visits over treatment control categories (4 being indicative of higher perception of treatment control).

Most of the bivariable associations noted between predictors and HSU in the overall group analysis (table 4a) were not consistently associated with HSU after stratification (tables 4b and 4c), suggesting some confounding (addressed above) and some effect measure modification by primary diagnosis. Therefore, the following associations are examined within the subgroups.

Among children with GDD (Table 4b), the primary enabling factor associated with increased HSU was parental employment (average 2 more annual visits per year), while the primary needs factor was a concurrent syndromic diagnosis (almost 2 more annual visits per year), although estimates had limited precision.

Among children with ASD, families who paid R100 or more per hospital visit on average attended 6 more annual visits (β 5.95, 95% CI 2.47 to 9.43, p=0.0001), suggesting an association with higher SES levels (enabling factor), which was also reflected in the higher number of annual visits associated with caregiver tertiary education (β 2.71, 95% CI 0.17 to 5.24, *p*=0.04). Girls with ASD attended 3 more annual visits per annum than boys (*p*=0.04), as did children whose caregiver reported CAM use (p=0.005), likely reflecting needs factors related to severity of the diagnosis. Several psycho-social factors were associated with HSU among families of children with ASD. Each 1unit increase in the Brief IPQ score for personal control was associated with 1 more annual visit (*p*=0.009), and for treatment control, just under 2 more annual visits (*p*<0.0001, table 4b). Similarly, a higher satisfaction score on the PSQ-18 patient satisfaction questionnaire predicted a greater number of health visits. By contrast, increasing scores on the brief family distress scale predicted lower HSU, with 1 fewer visit per annum per unit increase in the distress score (*p*=0.003).

(Other factors assessed in bivariate analyses that were not found significant are presented in Appendix 3).

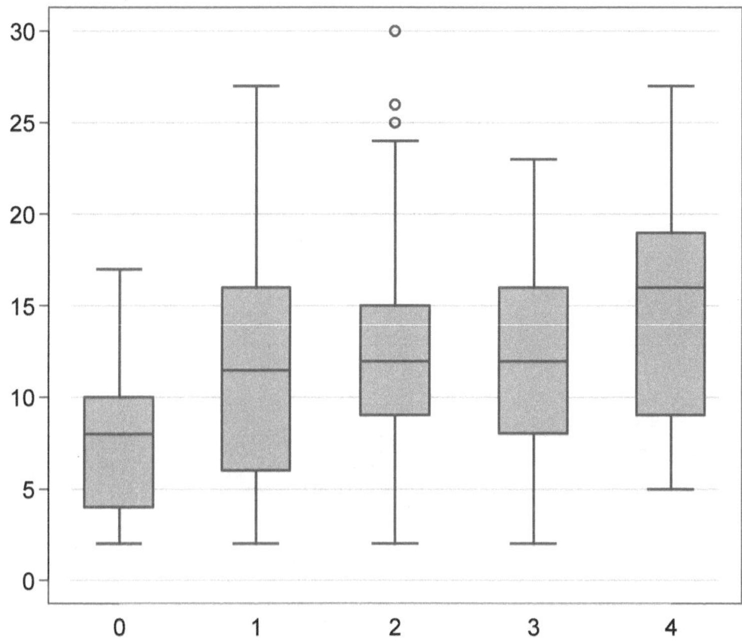


**Figure 4. Box-and-whiskers plots showing health care utilization over indicator for caregiver's perception of treatment control**

**TABLE 6. Factors associated with health care utilization (a) overall; (b) restricted to children with primary diagnosis of ASD; and (c) restricted to children with primary diagnosis of GDD: mean differences with 95% confidence intervals from linear regression**

| | (a) Full cohort (N=240) | | (b) Children with GDD (n=124) | | (c) Children with ASD (n=116) | |
|---|---|---|---|---|---|---|
| | Crude *β* coefficient (95% CI) | *p* | Crude *β* coefficient (95% CI) | *p* | Crude *β* coefficient (95% CI) | *p* |
| **NEED FACTORS** | | | | | | |
| Primary diagnosis | | | | | | |
| *GDD (ref)* | 1.00 | - | n/a | - | n/a | - |
| *ASD* | -1.76 (-3.20; -0.32) | 0.02 | n/a | - | n/a | - |
| Presence of genetic syndrome | | | | | | |
| *Non syndromic* | 1.00 | - | 1.00 | - | 1.00 | - |
| *Has a syndromic diagnosis* | 2.19 (0.50; 3.88) | 0.01 | 1.89 (-0.29; 4.07) | 0.09 | 1.14 (-2.18; 4.47) | 0.50 |
| Co-occurring morbidity | | | | | | |
| *No other known chronic diagnosis* | 1.00 | - | 1.00 | - | 1.00 | - |
| *≥1 other chronic diagnosis* | 0.95 (-0.68; 2.58) | 0.25 | 0.98 (-1.18; 3.14) | 0.37 | -1.23 (-4.22; 1.76) | 0.42 |
| Age at which child received primary diagnosis | | | | | | |
| *≥ 2 years of age* | 1.00 | - | 1.00 | - | 1.00 | - |
| *< 2 years of age* | 1.72 (0.26; 3.17) | 0.02 | 1.49 (-0.64; 3.62) | 0.17 | 1.15 (-0.98; 3.29) | 0.29 |
| Brief family distress scale | | | | | | |
| | -0.51 (-1.11; 0.09) | 0.09 | 0.10 (-0.78; 0.99) | 0.82 | -1.20 (-1.98; -0.41) | 0.003 |
| **ENABLING FACTORS** | | | | | | |
| Parental employment | | | | | | |
| *Neither parent is employed full-time (ref)* | 1.00 | - | 1.00 | - | 1.00 | - |
| *At least one parent is employed full-time* | 1.34 (-0.17; 2.85) | 0.08 | 2.05 (-0.27; 4.37) | 0.08 | 1.24 (-0.72; 3.20) | 0.21 |
| Cost of travelling to and from hospital | | | | | | |
| *<R100 (ref)* | 1.00 | | 1.00 | - | 1.00 | - |
| *≥ R100* | 4.19 (1.67; 6.71) | 0.001 | 2.66 (-0.92; 6.23) | 0.14 | 5.95 (2.47; 9.43) | 0.001 |

**TABLE 6 (continued)**

| | (a) Full cohort (N=240) | | (b) Children with GDD (n=124) | | (c) Children with ASD (n=116) | |
|---|---|---|---|---|---|---|
| | **Crude β coefficient (95% CI)** | ***p*** | **Crude β coefficient (95% CI)** | ***p*** | **Crude β coefficient (95% CI)** | ***p*** |
| Binary income indicator | | | | | | |
| *≥R8000/month (ref)* | 1.00 | - | 1.00 | - | 1.00 | - |
| *< R8000/month* | -0.93 (-3.13; 1.26) | 0.40 | -0.91 (-4.65; 2.84) | 0.63 | -1.47 (-4.09; 1.16) | 0.27 |
| **PREDISPOSING FACTORS** | | | | | | |
| Child sex | | | | | | |
| *Male* | 1.00 | - | 1.00 | - | 1.00 | - |
| *Female* | 1.59 (0.03; 3.14) | 0.04 | 0.63 (-1.56; 2.83) | 0.57 | 2.31 (0.10; 4.52) | 0.04 |
| Caregiver relationship status | | | | | | |
| *Single/unmarried (ref)* | 1.00 | - | 1.00 | - | 1.00 | - |
| *Married/co-habiting* | 1.61 (0.11-3.11) | 0.04 | 1.38 (-0.77; 3.54) | 0.21 | 2.31 (0.24-4.37) | 0.03 |
| Caregiver highest level of education | | | | | | |
| *Does not have tertiary education (ref)* | 1.00 | - | 1.00 | - | 1.00 | - |
| *Has tertiary education* | 0.26 (-1.78; 2.30) | 0.80 | -2.31 (-5.47; 0.84) | 0.15 | 2.71 (0.17; 5.24) | 0.04 |
| Caregiver reports of complementary or alternative medicines (CAM) | | | | | | |
| *No CAM use known* | 1.00 | - | 1.00 | - | 1.00 | - |
| *Known to use CAM* | 1.64 (0.03; 3.24) | 0.05 | 0.36 (-2.03; 2.75) | 0.76 | 3.02 (0.92; 5.11) | 0.005 |
| Brief illness perspective questionnaire (B-IPQ) | | | | | | |
| Personal control | 0.53 (-0.16; 1.23) | 0.13 | -0.27 (-1.35; 0.81) | 0.62 | 1.18 (0.30-2.05) | 0.009 |
| Treatment control | 1.07 (0.38; 1.76) | 0.003 | 0.14 (-0.94; 1.22) | 0.79 | 1.79 (0.94; 2.64) | <0.0001 |
| Patient satisfaction questionnaire (PSQ-18) | | | | | | |
| General satisfaction | 0.36 (-0.82; 1.55) | 0.55 | -0.64 (-2.11; 0.82) | 0.38 | 1.45 (-0.09; 2.99) | 0.06 |
| Satisfaction overall | 0.12 (-0.13; 0.37) | 0.35 | -0.06 (-0.42; 0.30) | 0.74 | 0.29 (-0.04; 0.62) | 0.09 |

Abbreviations: GDD, global developmental disorder; ASD, autism spectrum disorder; CI, confidence interval, Beta-coefficients represent mean difference in health care visits: comparing each category to the reference, or difference per unit increase for continuous variables

[1] *p*-value for interaction effect of indicated variable (e.g. child sex) with binary indicator for primary diagnosis (GDD vs ASD) is *p*<0.05, indicating likely presence of effect measure modification, i.e. *p*<0.05 suggests that the relationship between indicated variable and overall health care visits varies within subgroups of primary diagnosis

## TABLE 7. Health care utilization comparing children with primary diagnosis of ASD to those with primary diagnosis of GDD: adjusted mean differences with 95% confidence intervals from multivariable linear regression

| | **Adjusted *β* coefficient[1] (95% confidence interval)** | ***p*-value** |
|---|---|---|
| Primary diagnosis | | |
| *Global developmental disorder (ref)* | 1.00 | - |
| *Autism spectrum disorder* | -1.19 (-2.73; 0.36) | 0.13 |
| Parental employment | | |
| *Neither parent is employed full-time (ref)* | 1.00 | - |
| *At least one parent is employed full-time* | 1.49 (-0.02; 3.00) | 0.05 |
| Age at which child received primary diagnosis | | |
| *≥ 2 years of age* | 1.00 | - |
| *< 2 years of age* | 0.89 (-0.64; 2.43) | 0.25 |
| Child sex | | |
| *Male* | 1.00 | - |
| *Female* | 1.04 (-0.51; 2.60) | 0.19 |
| Presence of genetic syndrome | | |
| *Not diagnosed with syndrome* | 1.00 | - |
| *Has a syndromic diagnosis* | 1.43 (-0.38; 3.24) | 0.12 |

Abbreviations: GDD, global developmental disorder; ASD, autism spectrum disorder; beta-coefficients represent mean difference in health care visits comparing ASD to GDD (i.e. GDD – ASD)

[1] All variables included in the model are shown with coefficients and 95% confidence intervals

### 3.8 Unmet needs

Most caregivers were unable to reliably determine any specialist services that the child required but could not attend. To determine unmet therapy needs, therapy visits attended were subtracted from those recommended as the minimum standard of care for children receiving early intervention therapy in our service. Majority of the children required both speech and occupational therapy comprising maximum of 24 therapy visits. Both groups of children had similarly high proportions of unmet needs: 0.66 (SD 0.21) among those with ASD vs 0.69 (SD 0.21) among those with GDD, $p$=0.33 (Table 8).

**TABLE 8. Distribution of unmet therapy needs among all children and within sub-groups of children according to primary diagnosis**

| | Overall (N=240) | Global developmental delay (GDD, n=124) | Autism Spectrum disorder (ASD, n=116) | Difference in proportions (95% CI)[3] | *p*-value |
|---|---|---|---|---|---|
| Number of *recommended*[1] core therapy[2] visits (A) | 24 (2) | 24 (3) | 24 (2) | - | - |
| Number of *scheduled* (attended + missed) core therapy[2] visits (B) | 8 (5) | 7 (5) | 8 (5) | - | - |
| Number of visits[2] that were not offered (A-B) | 16 (5) | 17 (5) | 16 (5) | - | - |
| Proportion unmet needs (A-B)/(B) | 0.68 (0.22) | 0.69 (0.21) | 0.66 (0.21) | 0.03 (-0.03-0.08) | 0.33 |

Distributional values are mean (standard deviation); difference between means provided with 95% confidence intervals, CI with p-value calculated using t-test

1 Following best practices guideline (set as bi-monthly per child for both groups)

2 "Core therapy" defined as occupational therapy, physiotherapy and speech/language therapy using standard recommendations for primary diagnosis

3 Two-sample difference in proportion test (GDD – ASD)

Contributing to unmet therapy needs were missed appointments. About half of the children, 119/240 (49.6%) reported to have missed at least 1 booked therapy session (Table 9). The leading reasons cited for missed appointments included lack of transportation means (9.5%), commitment with other duties (9.2%), and lack of social support (9.2%).

**TABLE 9. Reasons provided for missing therapy visits among all children and within sub-groups of children according to primary diagnosis**

| | **Total (N=240)** | **Global Developmental Delay (n=124)** | **Autism Spectrum Disorder (n=116)** |
|---|---|---|---|
| Forgot | 11(4.6%) | 9(7.2%) | 2 (1.7%) |
| Commitment with other duties | 22 (9.2%) | 9(7.2%) | 13(11.2%) |
| Lack of transport means | 23(9.5%) | 12(9.7%) | 11(9.4%) |
| Lack of social support | 22(9.2%) | 8(6.5%) | 14(12.1%) |
| Child was unwell | 10(4.2%) | 5(4.0%) | 5(4.3%) |
| Bad weather | 5 (2.1%) | 1(0.8%) | 4(3.4%) |
| Problems at the facility | 13(5.4%) | 7(5.6%) | 6(5.8%) |
| Others | 13(5.4%) | 7(5.6%) | 6(5.8%) |
| **Total missed appointments** | 119(49.6%) | 58(46.8%) | 61(52.6%) |

# CHAPTER 4 DISCUSSION AND CONCLUSIONS

## 4.1 Discussion

The aim of this study was to compare HSU patterns of children with ASD and GDD attending services at a tertiary facility. Overall, the mean frequency of health care visits in this cohort was 12.4 visits per child per annum. We observed a higher service use among children with GDD (13.3) compared to those with ASD (11.5). This primarily reflected higher frequency of specialist visits in children with GDD VS ASD (4.0 vs 2.0), because of their higher comorbid diagnoses (41.0% vs 12.1%) and higher syndromic diagnoses (37.1% versus 9.5%). These findings differ from observations made in studies done in the USA which have demonstrated higher annual outpatient visits among children with ASD compared to those typically developing (42, 44), as well as those with other NDD across various services (86, 96). This included physician visits, psychiatric visits, and core therapy visits. One possible explanation to this variance stems from the fact that children with GDD recorded more multisystemic medical conditions, and congenital/genetic conditions than those with ASD, which necessitated more specialist consultations. Secondly, chronic illnesses may have contributed to their developmental delays. However, though presence of >1 documented comorbid condition was considered as a need variable, it was not a found to be a predictor of higher service when analysed overall, and specifically among children with either ASD or GDD. This was contrary to findings of study by Zukerman and colleagues (2017) in the USA which reported higher service use among those with severer illness (58).

Much lower frequency of comorbidities was reported in this cohort, and these comprised largely of medical conditions (27%) and congenital/ syndromic diagnoses (24%). Much fewer children had documented comorbid NDD, psychiatric or behavioural comorbidities. These findings again contradict various studies that have reported high comorbid conditions in children with ASD from low income countries. Springer and colleagues (2013) in SA reported a high prevalence of behavioural problems (89%) in children with ASD (40). Similarly, Mpaka and colleagues in the Congo also found high rates of comorbidities including epilepsy (72.5%) and ID (75.8%) among children with ASD, and especially the older children (39). Likewise,

Belhadj and colleagues (2006) examined Tunisian children with ASD and documented comorbid ID in over 60% of cases studied (76). Bakare and colleagues (2011) in Nigeria also documented associated comorbid ID, epilepsy and oculocutaneous albinism in children with ASD (164). Similarly, studies done in the USA, have reported high ADHD and GDD/ID in children with ASD, and high behavioural and psychiatric comorbidities (87-97%), which accounted for most of the specialist and ED visits (38, 84). The low prevalence of mental health problems in our study may have arisen from various factors. Firstly, our study focused on preschool aged children, where these conditions are more easily manageable, compared to older children. Secondly, the clinical diagnosis in this study was done retrospectively from medical records. Under-diagnosis by clinicians may have arisen due difficulties in identification of comorbid conditions in non- verbal children with ASD, because of the lack of appropriate diagnostic tools. Thirdly, reduced awareness and stigma around mental health diagnosis may have contributed to low concerns raised by caregivers, hence the diagnosis. This may also explain the lower specialist visits, that led to lower overall service use in the ASD group. There is need for clinicians to raise their index of suspicion of these non-physical comorbidities, and to develop local tools for screening of all children with ASD for comorbid NDD and mental before starting on treatments (80).

Overall, other predictors of HSU in this cohort included being female, younger age, concurrent syndromic diagnosis, but these did not remain significant after controlling for primary diagnosis, hence were considered as confounders that were predictive of GDD diagnosis. In this cohort, 64% of caregivers were either married or cohabiting, and this was similar in both groups. The caregiver being married or having a partner was associated with higher service use in ASD households, suggesting better family stability was associated with improved service use. One third of families (33%) reported having no social supporter to accompany them to the health facility, and this was higher (40%) among households of children with GDD. However, the lack of a social supporter was not found to predict lower service use. Various studies have made empirical observations of high separation/ divorce rates among families of children with ASD, largely due to increased emotional and financial the stress of caring for the child. However, study by Freedman and colleagues (2011) done in the USA did not find this to be true (165).

We observed lower specialist visits in those with ASD compared to GDD. This partly reflects the lower documented comorbid disorders in the ASD group but may also reflect unmet specialist visits in this group, arising from underdiagnosis of comorbidities. Similar findings were reported by Krauss and colleagues in the USA who observed that one third of children with ASD, compared to just one fifth of children with ID and one fifth of children with other special care needs reported experiencing problems accessing specialty medical care services (49). Improved identification of comorbid diagnoses may increase specialist referrals.

Overall, the mean annual emergency visits were 1.0(1.0-2.0) visit per year, and this was similar in both groups. This ED visit rate is however much lower compared to studies in USA that have reported greater ED visits, especially among ASD children (26, 102). Deavenport and colleagues (2015) in their study assessing factors associated with ED utilization, reported that children with ASD had 0.26 times more annual ED visits compared to non-ASD children (102). However, the leading causes ED visits from this cohort were respiratory infections and unspecified fevers, which is like what they found. USA based studies have also reported 1.2 times higher rates of accidents or injuries among children with ASD compared to those with GDD presenting to ED (99, 100). On the contrary, accidents accounted for only 8.7% of all ED visits in our study. It may be that minor injuries were handled at home and did not reach the health facilities. Likewise, mental, and behavioural problems accounted for only 5.7% of ED visits in this cohort. This is contrary to observations made in the USA, which reported high psychiatric presentation among ED visits in children with ASD (26, 34). Possible explanations to this include issues such as cultural perspectives of mental illness, beliefs around effectiveness of interventions offered, and reduced awareness of possible existing interventions. Other potential barriers in LMIC households include the fact that health care systems place more focus on “life threatening” or serious medical illnesses due to financial constraints.

The mean annual rate of therapy visits was 6.0 (2.0-10.0), and this again was similar in the ASD and GDD groups. Therapy often target core symptoms or co-morbidities, and low visits imply reduced intensity of therapy for these children. Furthermore, we noted a large disparity in number of therapy services accessed per child, with up to 15% of children not receiving any therapy in the preceding year, yet the highest attended had 18 sessions in the year. Higher annual outpatient rates have been observed in USA based studies, in children with ASD, with some exceeding 41 visits per child per annum (42), and therapy formed the largest proportion of these outpatient visits. This low therapy uptake can be attributed to low importance attributed to therapy by households, or to limited access to therapy services (54). The latter is further supported by the fact that 68% of children in this cohort reported unmet therapy needs in this cohort. There has been a growing demand for therapy services, especially in urban areas, that has overstretched available capacity. However, demand for service does not always translate to utilization. Research has shown that contextual factors such as organizational features or provider characteristics may contribute to limited utilization (53). Most children in this study accessed therapy at CDH. Inefficiency, due to limited number of trained personnel and other resources may discourage service use in these primary level centres. This is further supported by the low parent ratings of their previous experiences in respect to the physical environment, and facility management of disruptive behaviour at CHD. In addition, areas of service dissatisfaction as reported by parents included accessibility and convenience, and limited time spent with health providers. The World Health Organization (WHO) recommends provision of EIT in the child's naturalistic environments, either through home-based care or at nearest community rehabilitation centres. This offers 3 advantages, as it allows caregivers to work in familiar environments, reduces time and travel costs, and maintains the family unit. Community service should be accessible, affordable, acceptable, equitable, efficient, and sustainable. Therapy access could be improved by better systemic structuring, re-organization of therapy programs to reduce inconvenience to families, promotion of group therapy sessions to bridge the demand gaps and building of capacity.

Because of lack of practise guidelines on intensity of interventions for the various NDD locally, most facilities strive to provide at least 1 session per discipline per month as the routine standard of care. Children therefore receive varying intensity of EIP depending on the facility attended, and availability of therapists. We found similar therapy visits in children with ASD as in those with GDD. On the contrary, some studies have observed that children with ASD receive the lowest quality of care of all CWSN (166). Contributors have included sociodemographic characteristics of families (65, 167), condition severity (166), and complexity of care needs (38, 166). ASD children that receive high quality care, both they and their families may have improved health outcomes and functional status (62). Lack of practice guidelines prevents facilities from optimizing individual therapy needs to meet the child's needs, and parents from demanding better services for their children, during this narrow window of opportunity, when EIP makes the greatest impact on outcomes.

Primary care is important for disease prevention, health promotion and monitoring of children health in general. The recommended frequency of primary care visits for children between 3-5 years is biannually, and annually thereafter. In addition to other scheduled childhood vaccinations, the World Health Organization (WHO) also recommends yearly flu vaccination for children with NDD. In this cohort, 73% were up to date on immunizations, but only 42.9% had attended at least 1 primary visit in the preceding year. It means that most children did not attend any primary care services after completing their primary immunizations. This therefore suggests suboptimal primary care for this group, despite their numerous health encounters. Similar observations were observed by Cummings and colleagues (2016) who observed that children with ASD were less likely to receive preventive services. On the contrary, other studies in developed countries observed either no difference (60), or slightly higher (63) attendance rates in primary care visits between ASD compared to non-ASD children. The high pressure on caregivers to attend other services may make them forgo primary care visits. This could be minimised by integrating all services needed, to reduce inconvenience to caregivers.

Health financing is an enabling factor, and low family income often poses a barrier to health service access globally (59, 86). Though households with children with ASD had higher parent employment rates compared to those with GDD (42% vs 29%), overall, most (87%) households in this cohort had a net family income of <R8000 per month. Controlling for other confounders, households with children with ASD, who spent > R100 per hospital visit, attended 6 more annual visits. This also reflected the higher number of annual visits associated with caregiver tertiary education. On multivariable analysis, parental employment emerged as the strongest residual predictive factor for increased service use. Similar findings were reported by Irvin and colleagues (2012), who observed that higher SES was associated with receiving more services (105). Efforts to improve HSU in low resourced countries have focused on elimination of financial barriers to access, by making service free in children. However, medical expenses typically make up only a small portion of overall spending by families caring for children with special needs (168). Non-medical expenses covering transportation costs, modifications to houses, specialized childcare, and special food, clothing, and other items, can cause huge financial burdens on families. Spending on these out-of-pocket medical expenses may drive household to experience catastrophic economic burden and fall into poverty, denying then access. Removing financial hardships is particularly crucial for developing countries where out-of-pocket is the main payment strategy for health care. This could be mitigated by provision of the child support grants, and by designing programs that optimize care, but containing out-of-pocket costs.

HSU is largely consumer oriented, and uptake is subject level of knowledge, experiences, and perceptions of illness. To achieve optimal utilization of services, we need to enlist cooperation of caregivers. Qualitative assessment on illness perceptions found similarities in both ASD and GDD groups. The lowest perspective ratings were observed in two dimensions; treatment control and understanding of illness. Overall, caregiver belief that therapy was able to control illness and that the caregiver had personal control over the illness ($p<0.001$), predicted higher HSU. Similar observations were reported in a study done in France which demonstrated correlation between parental beliefs around the cause of illness and service use (117). On the other hand, in study done in the USA, caregiver belief in environmental causes was associated with receiving >20hr per week of ASD- related therapy per week (118). Parents face difficulties understanding these conditions, and this makes them resort to CAM use. One third (27.9%) of families in this cohort reported CAM use. This was similar in both ASD and GDD groups. Similar observations were made in the USA by Chadeiz and colleagues (2018) who observed that believe in environmental exposures, vaccines and medication as the cause for ASD, was associated with high

CAM use (118). On the other hand, in study by Zukerman and colleagues (2017), high CAM use was reported in households with no knowledge of aetiology, and those with severer illness (94). We observed higher HSU among households of children with ASD, whose caregivers reported CAM use, likely reflecting need factors related to severity of the diagnosis. On the contrary, Levy and colleagues (2010), documented high CAM use in families that had delay in diagnosis, delay in onset of EIP, or when access to conventional care was limited (35). Akins and colleagues (2014), observed similar findings of high CAM use among those with the most intensive therapy and those with higher education (96). Therefore, clinicians need to openly discuss CAM use with clients to allow informed decision making.

The level of family distress was found to be similar in both groups, however, in households with children with ASD, each 1unit increase in the 'Brief IPQ score' for personal control was associated with 1 more annual visit. This concurs with findings from study by Thomas and colleagues (2007) done in the USA, where parental mental health predicted increased ED use in families with ASD children (104). Similar findings were reported by studies done in Canada by Lunsky and colleagues (2012, 2017), they observed higher ED attendance by families of adolescents and adults with ASD experiencing distress (138, 139). In this study, there was however low linkage to auxiliary services such as family counsellors, despite their role in supporting families in distress. Brief family distress measures can assist clinicians to determine those needing more interventions (157).

The overall satisfaction level was 68.3%, with highest rating in communication and technical quality. However, clients expressed some dissatisfaction with the physical environment, which was largely related to disruptive behaviours arising from the overstimulating hospital environments in waiting area. Some caregivers also felt that instructions provided for home therapy were inadequate. USA based studies have reported significant dissatisfaction among households of children with ASD experiencing less collaboration, more disagreements and more dissatisfaction with services received (64, 65), reflecting poor partnerships with their service providers.

Ratings of experiences were similar in both groups. In households with ASD, higher satisfaction score predicted a greater number of health visits. Overall, satisfaction level was quite favourable, but the few areas of dissatisfaction need to be improved. Clients' experience and opinions are important in improving health care services, shaping health policies, and providing feedback on the quality, availability, and responsiveness of health care services.

In our study, the mean overall hospitalization rate was 22.5% per annum, but we observed a higher hospitalization rate in those with GDD, compared to the ASD group (31% vs 14%). Much higher hospitalization rates were observed in our study compared to studies in high income countries. Birenbaum and colleagues (1990) in the USA reported 10% annual hospitalization rates in children with ASD compared to 3% among those typically developing (169). On the other hand, Arim and colleagues (2017) in Canada found that children with NDD had three times more hospitalizations than typically developing children (41). The higher hospitalizations rates in our study reflected the multimorbidity diagnoses in the GDD group, but could also be a reflection of the higher prevalence of community based infectious diseases.

## 4.2 Conclusions

Children with GDD had greater HSU compared to those with ASD, primarily due to their higher specialist visits, because of higher prevalence of syndromic and comorbid chronic conditions. Overall, a low intensity of core therapy was observed in both groups, with majority not meeting the stipulated routine standard of care, reflecting high proportion of unmet therapy needs. Missed appointments also contributed to this. Health satisfaction level was favourable in both ASD and GDD households, but dissatisfaction was mainly reported in the time spent with health providers and accessibility and convenience of services. Low level of satisfaction predicted lower service use in households with children with ASD. Children from lower socioeconomic backgrounds were associated with reduced health service use. Having either parent in employment was the largest predictors of high service use. One third of households were using CAM therapies. Among households with children with ASD, use of CAM therapy as was associated with higher service use, reflecting perceived severity, a need factor. We observed similar rates of family distress in families with children with ASD and GDD, but high level of family distress predicted HSU among households with children with ASD.

## 4.3 Recommendations

All services were generally underutilized. To minimize serve access disparities, future programs need to bridge financial access barriers by adopting strategies that can reduce out-of-pocket costs, such as provision of accessible and efficient community-based programs, and through improved caregiver education on effective interventions. There is need to develop local clinical practise guidelines that target to optimise intensity of core therapy, to enable service providers and caregivers to adequately plan for these services, and therefore improve compliance. There is need to improve the recognition of comorbid mental and medical diagnoses among children with ASD, by raising the clinician's index of suspicion and developing culturally sensitive diagnostic tools will allow early intervention and institution of coordinated multidisciplinary services required by these children. Facilities need to implement client-oriented care, that focus on improving client experiences and level of satisfaction, by optimizing provider-patient contact time, and minimizing inconveniences caused to caregivers. This can strengthen the parent-professional-partnerships, improve care collaboration, and encourage open dialogue on CAM therapies. Providers should strive to recognize the family distress level among children with NDD, and subsequently link them to existing support services, as this may reduce unnecessary health service use.

## 4.4 Future research

There are several knowledge gaps on HSU in children with NDD that remain unanswered. There is need for a large multicentre prospective study, that can comprehensively quantify all the health service needs, unmet needs, and health service usage among these children. There is also need for a comprehensive assessment of out of pocket costs in care access for children with NDD, which will guide service planning and budgeting. Our study did not evaluate the how caregiver level of knowledge and stigma impacts on HSU among these children. The tools used to assess qualitative measures including perceptions, level of satisfaction, and family distress level, have all been validated in high income countries. There is need to assess the reliability and validity of these questionnaires in assessment of these variables in low income settings. Many participants required some assistance to complete the 12-page questionnaire, and others perceived the questions on experiences and on the level of satisfaction overlap significantly. Their adaptation to the local settings may be useful for future studies. There is need to develop better screening tools to evaluate comorbid mental, behavioural, and cognitive problems among preschool children with NDD in low income countries.

### 4.5 Limitations

There were 3 areas of potential sources of selection bias; Firstly, the study was done at a tertiary centre and therefore may not be representative of those attending private facilities, or those not accessing any services. Secondly, children referred to tertiary services are likely to be those with more severer problems, and multisystemic comorbidities. Thirdly, caregivers of severely affected children with ASD, were less likely to be included, as they unlikely to consent to participation in a 30-minute interview due to their behavioural challenges. Recall bias was inevitable from need for caregivers to recount events in the previous year, as underreporting of medical events increases over time. Emotional status of respondents at time of study may influence encoding and recall of events. Attendance to CDH was dependant on the record on the appointment card and patient recall and may have missed some visits that may have not been documented on the card. In this retrospective cohort design, the establishment of the primary diagnosis, and comorbid diagnoses in the children relied largely on a previous assessment, as documented in their medical records, and corroborated by parent reports. The diagnoses were not further validated by re-assessments of children in this cohort. This may explain the limited description of comorbid mental health and NDD problems commonly seen in ASD. On the other hand, the physical comorbidities were more likely to be captured among children with GDD. As such, segregation based on the mental comorbidities were too few to allow for a meaningful analysis, which may partly explain low specialist visits in ASD group.

# REFFRENCES

1. Association AP. Diagnostic and statistical manual of mental disorders (DSM-5®): American Psychiatric Pub; 2013.
2. Ozonoff S, Heung K, Byrd R, Hansen R, Hertz-Picciotto I. The onset of autism: Patterns of symptom emergence in the first years of Life. Autism research : official journal of the International Society for Autism Research. 2008;1(6):320-8.
3. Bolton PF, Golding J, Emond A, Steer CD. Autism Spectrum Disorder and autistic traits in the Avon Longitudinal Study of Parents and Children: Precursors and Early Signs. Journal of the American Academy of Child & Adolescent Psychiatry. 2012;51(3):249-60.e25.
4. Matson JL, Kozlowski AM. The increasing prevalence of autism spectrum disorders. Research in Autism Spectrum Disorders. 2011;5(1):418-25.
5. Elsabbagh M, Divan G, Koh Y-J, Kim YS, Kauchali S, Marcín C, et al. Global prevalence of autism and other pervasive developmental disorders. Autism Research. 2012;5(3):160-79.
6. Zablotsky B, Black LI, Maenner MJ, Schieve LA, Blumberg SJ. Estimated prevalence of autism and other developmental disabilities following questionnaire changes in the 2014 National Health Interview Survey. 2015.
7. Newschaffer CJ, Croen LA, Daniels J, Giarelli E, Grether JK, Levy SE, et al. The epidemiology of autism spectrum disorders. Annual review of public health. 2007;28:235-58.
8. Autism, Developmental Disabilities Monitoring Network Surveillance Year Principal I. Prevalence of Autism Spectrum Disorders — Autism and Developmental Disabilities Monitoring Network, 14 Sites, United States, 2008. Morbidity and Mortality Weekly Report: Surveillance Summaries. 2012;61(3):1-19.
9. Christianson A, Zwane M, Manga P, Rosen E, Venter A, Downs D, et al. Children with intellectual disability in rural South Africa: prevalence and associated disability. Journal of Intellectual Disability Research. 2002;46(2):179-86.
10. Giarelli E, Clarke DL, Catching C, Ratcliffe SJ. Developmental disabilities and behavioral problems among school children in the Western Cape of South Africa. Research in developmental disabilities. 2009;30(6):1297-305.
11. Reichow B. Overview of Meta-Analyses on Early Intensive Behavioral Intervention for young children with Autism Spectrum Disorders. Journal of Autism and Developmental Disorders. 2012;42(4):512-20.
12. Eldevik S, Hastings RP, Hughes JC, Jahr E, Eikeseth S, Cross S. Meta-analysis of early intensive behavioral intervention for children with autism. Journal of Clinical Child & Adolescent Psychology. 2009;38(3):439-50.
13. Weitlauf AS, McPheeters ML, Peters B, Sathe N, Travis R, Aiello R, et al. Therapies for children with autism spectrum disorder. Agency for healthcare Research and quality publication, No 14-EHC036-EF, August 2014
14. Howlin P, Magiati I, Charman T. Systematic review of early intensive behavioral interventions for children with autism. American journal on intellectual and developmental disabilities. 2009;114(1):23-41.
15. Copeland L, Buch G. Early intervention issues in autism spectrum disorders. Autism : the international journal of research and practice. 2013;3(109):2-7.
16. Levy SE, Hyman SL. Complementary and alternative medicine treatments for children with autism spectrum disorders. Child and adolescent psychiatric clinics of North America. 2008;17(4):803-20.
17. Strickland BB, Jones JR, Newacheck PW, Bethell CD, Blumberg SJ, Kogan MD. Assessing systems quality in a changing health care environment: The 2009–10 National Survey of Children with Special Health Care Needs. Maternal and child health journal. 2015;19(2):353-61.

18. Hong M, Lee SY, Han J, Park JC, Lee YJ, Hwangbo R, et al. Prescription trends of psychotropics in children and adolescents with Autism Based on Nationwide Health Insurance Data. Journal of Korean medical science. 2017;32(10):1687-93.
19. Lake JK, Weiss JA, Dergal J, Lunsky Y. Child, parent, and service predictors of psychotropic polypharmacy among adolescents and young adults with an autism spectrum disorder. Journal of child and adolescent psychopharmacology. 2014;24(9):486-93.
20. Mandell DS, Morales KH, Marcus SC, Stahmer AC, Doshi J, Polsky DE. Psychotropic medication use among Medicaid-enrolled children with autism spectrum disorders. Pediatrics. 2008;121(3):e441-8.
21. Jobski K, Hofer J, Hoffmann F, Bachmann C. Use of psychotropic drugs in patients with autism spectrum disorders: a systematic review. Acta psychiatrica Scandinavica. 2017;135(1):8-28.
22. Nath D. Complementary and Alternative Medicine in the School-Age Child With Autism. Journal of pediatric health care : official publication of National Association of Pediatric Nurse Associates & Practitioners. 2017;31(3):393-7.
23. Hall SE, Riccio CA. Complementary and alternative treatment use for autism spectrum disorders. Complementary therapies in clinical practice. 2012;18(3):159-63.
24. Louw K-A. Prevalence and patterns of medication use in children and adolescents with autism spectrum disorders in the Western Cape: book, University of Cape Town; 2012.
25. Schieve LA, Gonzalez V, Boulet SL, Visser SN, Rice CE, Van Naarden Braun K, et al. Concurrent medical conditions and health care use and needs among children with learning and behavioral developmental disabilities, National Health Interview Survey, 2006-2010. Research in developmental disabilities. 2012;33(2):467-76.
26. Iannuzzi DA, Cheng ER, Broder-Fingert S, Bauman ML. Brief report: Emergency department utilization by individuals with autism. J Autism Dev Disord. 2015;45(4):1096-102.
27. Vohra R, Madhavan S, Sambamoorthi U. Comorbidity prevalence, healthcare utilization, and expenditures of Medicaid enrolled adults with autism spectrum disorders. Autism : the international journal of research and practice. 2017;21(8):995-1009.
28. Cohen-Silver JH, Muskat B, Ratnapalan S. Autism in the emergency department. Clinical pediatrics. 2014;53(12):1134-8.
29. Simonoff E, Pickles A, Charman T, Chandler S, Loucas T, Baird G. Psychiatric Disorders in Children With Autism Spectrum Disorders: Prevalence, Comorbidity, and Associated Factors in a Population-Derived Sample. Journal of the American Academy of Child & Adolescent Psychiatry. 2008;47(8):921-9.
30. Gillberg C. The ESSENCE in child psychiatry: early symptomatic syndromes eliciting neurodevelopmental clinical examinations. Research in developmental disabilities. 2010;31(6):1543-51.
31. Joshi G, Petty C, Wozniak J, Henin A, Fried R, Galdo M, et al. The heavy burden of psychiatric comorbidity in youth with autism spectrum disorders: A large comparative study of a psychiatrically referred population. Journal of autism and developmental disorders. 2010;40(11):1361-70.
32. Leyfer OT, Folstein SE, Bacalman S, Davis NO, Dinh E, Morgan J, et al. Comorbid psychiatric disorders in children with autism: interview development and rates of disorders. Journal of autism and developmental disorders. 2006;36(7):849-61.
33. Croen LA, Zerbo O, Qian Y, Massolo ML, Rich S, Sidney S, et al. The health status of adults on the autism spectrum. Autism : the international journal of research and practice. 2015;19(7):814-23.
34. Kalb LG, Stuart EA, Freedman B, Zablotsky B, Vasa R. Psychiatric-related emergency department visits among children with an autism spectrum disorder. Pediatric Emergency Care. 2012;28(12):1269-76.
35. Levy SE, Giarelli E, Lee L-C, Schieve LA, Kirby RS, Cunniff C, et al. Autism Spectrum Disorder and Co-occurring Developmental, Psychiatric, and Medical Conditions Among Children in Multiple

Populations of the United States. Journal of Developmental & Behavioral Pediatrics. 2010;31(4):267-75.
36. Fombonne E. Epidemiology of pervasive developmental disorders. Pediatric research. 2009;65(6):591.
37. McPheeters M, Davis A, Navarre J, Scott T. Family Report of ASD Concomitant with Depression or Anxiety Among US Children. Journal of Autism & Developmental Disorders. 2011;41(5):646-53.
38. Ahmedani BK, Hock RM. Health care access and treatment for children with co-morbid autism and psychiatric conditions. Social psychiatry and psychiatric epidemiology. 2012;47(11):1807-14.
39. Mpaka DM, Okitundu DL, Ndjukendi AO, N'Situ A M, Kinsala SY, Mukau JE, et al. Prevalence and comorbidities of autism among children referred to the outpatient clinics for neurodevelopmental disorders. The Pan African medical journal. 2016;25:82.
40. Springer PE, van Toorn R, Laughton B, Kidd M. Characteristics of children with pervasive developmental disorders attending a developmental clinic in the Western Cape Province, South Africa. South African Journal of Child Health. 2013;7(3):95-9.
41. Arim RG, Miller AR, Guèvremont A, Lach LM, Brehaut JC, Kohen DE. Children with neurodevelopmental disorders and disabilities: a population-based study of healthcare service utilization using administrative data. Developmental Medicine & Child Neurology. 2017;59(12):1284-90.
42. Liptak GS, Stuart T, Auinger P. Health care utilization and expenditures for children with autism: data from U.S. national samples. J Autism Dev Disord. 2006;36(7):871-9.
43. Vohra R, Madhavan S, Sambamoorthi U, St Peter C. Access to services, quality of care, and family impact for children with autism, other developmental disabilities, and other mental health conditions. Autism : the international journal of research and practice. 2013;18(7):815-26.
44. Croen LA, Najjar DV, Ray GT, Lotspeich L, Bernal P. A comparison of health care utilization and costs of children with and without autism spectrum disorders in a large group-model health plan. Pediatrics. 2006;118(4):e1203-11.
45. Peacock G, Amendah D, Ouyang L, Grosse SD. Autism spectrum disorders and health care expenditures: the effects of co-occurring conditions. Journal of Developmental & Behavioral Pediatrics. 2012;33(1):2-8.
46. Lee L-C, Harrington RA, Louie BB, Newschaffer CJ. Children with autism: Quality of life and parental concerns. Journal of autism and developmental disorders. 2008;38(6):1147-60.
47. Ambikile JS, Outwater A. Challenges of caring for children with mental disorders: Experiences and views of caregivers attending the outpatient clinic at Muhimbili National Hospital, Dar es Salaam - Tanzania. Child and Adolescent Psychiatry and Mental Health. 2012;6(1):16.
48. Bonis S. Stress and Parents of Children with Autism: A Review of Literature. Issues in Mental Health Nursing. 2016;37(3):153-63.
49. Krauss MW, Gulley S, Sciegaj M, Wells N. Access to specialty medical care for children with mental retardation, autism, and other special health care needs. Mental retardation. 2003;41(5):329-39.
50. Benevides T, Carretta H, Lane S. Unmet need for therapy among children with Autism Spectrum Disorder: Results from the 2005-2006 and 2009-2010 National Survey of Children with Special Health Care Needs. Maternal & Child Health Journal. 2016;20(4):878-88.
51. Warfield ME, Gulley S. Unmet need and problems accessing specialty medical and related services among children with special health care needs. Maternal and child health journal. 2006;10(2):201-16.
52. Kogan MD, Newacheck PW, Honberg L, Strickland B. Association between underinsurance and access to care among children with special health care needs in the United States. Pediatrics. 2005;116(5):1162-9.

53. Chiri G, Warfield M. Unmet need and problems accessing core health care services for children with Autism Spectrum Disorder. Maternal & Child Health Journal. 2012;16(5):1081-91.
54. Saloojee G, Phohole M, Saloojee H, IJsselmuiden C. Unmet health, welfare and educational needs of disabled children in an impoverished South African peri-urban township. Child: care, health and development. 2007;33(3):230-5.
55. Redfern A. An analysis of the prevalence of children with disabilities and disabling chronic illnesses in Western Health subdistrict of Cape Town, and the services available to them. University of Cape Town. 2014;book_hsf_2014_redfern_aw.pdf.
56. Andersen RM. Revisiting the behavioral model and access to medical care: does it matter? Journal of health and social behavior. 1995:1-10.
57. Boulet SL, Boyle CA, Schieve LA. Health care use and health and functional impact of developmental disabilities among US children, 1997-2005. Archives of pediatrics & adolescent medicine. 2009;163(1):19-26.
58. Zuckerman KE, Friedman NDB, Chavez AE, Shui AM, Kuhlthau KA. Parent-Reported severity and Health/Educational services use among US children with Autism: Results from a National Survey. Journal of developmental and behavioral pediatrics : JDBP. 2017;38(4):260-8.
59. Nguyen CT, Krakowiak P, Hansen R, Hertz-Picciotto I, Angkustsiri K. Sociodemographic Disparities in Intervention Service Utilization in Families of Children with Autism Spectrum Disorder. J Autism Dev Disord. 2016;46(12):3729-38.
60. Cummings JR, Lynch FL, Rust KC, Coleman KJ, Madden JM, Owen-Smith AA, et al. Health Services Utilization among Children with and without Autism Spectrum Disorders. Journal of Autism and Developmental Disorders. 2016;46(3):910-20.
61. DePape A-M, Lindsay S. Parents' Experiences of Caring for a Child With Autism Spectrum Disorder. Qualitative Health Research. 2014;25(4):569-83.
62. Kogan MD, Strickland BB, Blumberg SJ, Singh GK, Perrin JM, van Dyck PC. A national profile of the health care experiences and family impact of autism spectrum disorder among children in the United States, 2005-2006. Pediatrics. 2008;122(6):e1149-58.
63. Gurney JG, McPheeters ML, Davis MM. Parental report of health conditions and health care use among children with and without autism: National Survey of Children's Health. Archives of pediatrics & adolescent medicine. 2006;160(8):825-30.
64. Wilson SA, Peterson CC. Medical care experiences of children with autism and their parents: A scoping review. Child: care, health and development. 2018;44(6):807-17.
65. Liptak GS, Benzoni LB, Mruzek DW, Nolan KW, Thingvoll MA, Wade CM, et al. Disparities in diagnosis and access to health services for children with autism: data from the National Survey of Children's Health. Journal of developmental and behavioral pediatrics : JDBP. 2008;29(3):152-60.
66. Myers SM, Johnson CP. Management of children with autism spectrum disorders. Pediatrics. 2007;120(5):1162-82.
67. Council NR. Educating children with autism: National Academies Press; 2001.
68. Volkmar FR, Wiesner LA, Westphal A. Healthcare issues for children on the autism spectrum. Current opinion in psychiatry. 2006;19(4):361-6.
69. Chambers JG, Shkolnik J, Perez M. Total expenditures for students with disabilities, 1999-2000: Spending Variation by Disability. Report. Special Education Expenditure Project (SEEP). 2003.
70. Johnson E, Hastings RP. Facilitating factors and barriers to the implementation of intensive home-based behavioural intervention for young children with autism. Child: care, health and development. 2002;28(2):123-9.
71. Mouridsen S, Rich B, Isager T. Psychiatric disorders in adults diagnosed as children with atypical autism. A case control study. Journal of neural transmission. 2008;115(1):135-8.

72. Matson JL, Wilkins J, Macken J. The relationship of challenging behaviors to severity and symptoms of autism spectrum disorders. Journal of Mental Health Research in Intellectual Disabilities. 2008;2(1):29-44.
73. Horovitz M, Matson JL, Rieske RD, Kozlowski AM, Sipes M. The relationship between race and challenging behaviours in infants and toddlers with autistic disorder and pervasive developmental disorder–not otherwise specified. Developmental Neurorehabilitation. 2011;14(4):208-14.
74. Mayes SD, Calhoun SL. Impact of IQ, age, SES, gender, and race on autistic symptoms. Research in Autism Spectrum Disorders. 2011;5(2):749-57.
75. Mandell DS, Walrath CM, Manteuffel B, Sgro G, Pinto-Martin J. Characteristics of children with autistic spectrum disorders served in comprehensive community-based mental health settings. J Autism Dev Disord. 2005;35(3):313-21.
76. Belhadj A, Mrad R, Halayem M. A clinic and a paraclinic study of Tunisian population of children with autism. About 63 cases. La Tunisie Medicale. 2006;84(12):763-7.
77. Minshawi NF, Hurwitz S, Morriss D, McDougle CJ. Multidisciplinary assessment and treatment of self-injurious behavior in autism spectrum disorder and intellectual disability: integration of psychological and biological theory and approach. Journal of autism and developmental disorders. 2015;45(6):1541-68.
78. Isaksen J, Bryn V, Diseth TH, Heiberg A, Schjølberg S, Skjeldal OH. Children with autism spectrum disorders–the importance of medical investigations. European Journal of Paediatric Neurology. 2013;17(1):68-76.
79. Antshel KM, Polacek C, McMahon M, Dygert K, Spenceley L, Dygert L, et al. Comorbid ADHD and anxiety affect social skills group intervention treatment efficacy in children with autism spectrum disorders. Journal of Developmental & Behavioral Pediatrics. 2011;32(6):439-46.
80. Gadow KD, DeVincent C, Schneider J. Predictors of psychiatric symptoms in children with an autism spectrum disorder. Journal of autism and developmental Disorders. 2008;38(9):1710-20.
81. Mandell DS. Psychiatric hospitalization among children with autism spectrum disorders. Journal of autism and developmental disorders. 2008;38(6):1059-65.
82. Stark KH, Barnes JC, Young ND, Gabriels RL. Brief report: understanding crisis behaviors in hospitalized psychiatric patients with autism spectrum disorder—iceberg assessment interview. Journal of autism and developmental disorders. 2015;45(11):3468-74.
83. Mire SS, Raff NS, Brewton CM, Goin-Kochel RP. Age-related trends in treatment use for children with autism spectrum disorder. Research in Autism Spectrum Disorders. 2015;15:29-41.
84. Zablotsky B, Pringle BA, Colpe LJ, Kogan MD, Rice C, Blumberg SJ. Service and treatment use among children diagnosed with autism spectrum disorders. Journal of developmental and behavioral pediatrics : JDBP. 2015;36(2):98-105.
85. Atladóttir H, Schendel D, Lauritsen M, Henriksen T, Parner E. Patterns of contact with hospital for children with an Autism Spectrum Disorder: A Danish Register-Based Study. Journal of Autism & Developmental Disorders. 2012;42(8):1717-28.
86. Tregnago MK, Cheak-Zamora NC. Systematic review of disparities in health care for individuals with autism spectrum disorders in the United States. Research in Autism Spectrum Disorders. 2012;6(3):1023-31.
87. Huang ZJ, Kogan MD, Stella MY, Strickland B. Delayed or forgone care among children with special health care needs: an analysis of the 2001 National Survey of Children with Special Health Care Needs. Ambulatory Pediatrics. 2005;5(1):60-7.
88.Grover V, Cooke J, Hollingshead J, Rip M. Facilities for the mentally handicapped in the Western Cape. Some pressing needs. South African medical journal= Suid-Afrikaanse tydskrif vir geneeskunde. 1987;71(2):85-7.

89. Lin SC, Yu SM. Disparities in Healthcare Access and Utilization among Children with Autism Spectrum Disorder from Immigrant Non-English Primary Language Households in the United States. International journal of MCH and AIDS. 2015;3(2):159-67.
90. Ruble LA, Heflinger CA, Renfrew JW, Saunders RC. Access and service use by children with autism spectrum disorders in Medicaid Managed Care. J Autism Dev Disord. 2005;35(1):3-13.
91. Thomas KC, Morrissey JP, McLaurin C. Use of autism-related services by families and children. J Autism Dev Disord. 2007;37(5):818-29.
92. Broder-Fingert S, Shui A, Pulcini CD, Kurowski D, Perrin JM. Racial and ethnic differences in subspecialty service use by children with autism. Pediatrics. 2013;132(1):94-100.
93. Volden J, Duku E, Shepherd C, Ba, Georgiades S, Bennett T, et al. Service utilization in a sample of preschool children with autism spectrum disorder: A Canadian snapshot. Paediatrics & child health. 2015;20(8):e43-7.
94. Zuckerman K, Lindly OJ, Chavez AE. Timeliness of Autism Spectrum Disorder diagnosis and use of services among U.S. elementary school-aged children. Psychiatric services (Washington, DC). 2017;68(1):33-40.
95. Peng C-Z, Hatlestad P, Klug MG, Kerbeshian J, Burd L. Health care costs and utilization rates for children with pervasive developmental disorders in North Dakota from 1998 to 2004: Impact on Medicaid. Journal of Child Neurology. 2009;24(2):140-7.
96. Akins RS, Krakowiak P, Angkustsiri K, Hertz-Picciotto I, Hansen RL. Utilization patterns of conventional and complementary/alternative treatments in children with autism spectrum disorders and developmental disabilities in a population-based study. Journal of developmental and behavioral pediatrics : JDBP. 2014;35(1):1-10.
97. Nageswaran S, Parish SL, Rose RA, Grady MD. Do children with developmental disabilities and mental health conditions have greater difficulty using health services than children with physical disorders? Maternal and child health journal. 2011;15(5):634-41.
98. Schlenz AM, Carpenter LA, Bradley C, Charles J, Boan A. Age Differences in Emergency Department Visits and Inpatient Hospitalizations in Preadolescent and Adolescent Youth with Autism Spectrum Disorders. Journal of Autism and Developmental Disorders. 2015;45(8):2382-91.
99. McDermott S, Zhou L, Mann J. Injury treatment among children with autism or pervasive developmental disorder. J Autism Dev Disord. 2008;38(4):626-33.
100. Kalb LG, Vasa RA, Ballard ED, Woods S, Goldstein M, Wilcox HC. Epidemiology of injury-related emergency department visits in the US among youth with autism spectrum disorder. Journal of autism and developmental disorders. 2016;46(8):2756-63.
101. Weiss JA, Tint A, Paquette-Smith M, Lunsky Y. Perceived self-efficacy in parents of adolescents and adults with autism spectrum disorder. Autism : the international journal of research and practice. 2016;20(4):425-34.
102. Deavenport-Saman A, Lu Y, Smith K, Yin L. Do Children with autism overutilize the emergency department? Examining visit urgency and subsequent hospital admissions. Maternal and child health journal. 2016;20(2):306-14.
103. Cidav Z, Lawer L, Marcus S, Mandell D. Age-related variation in health service use and associated expenditures among children with autism. Journal of Autism & Developmental Disorders. 2013;43(4):924-31.
104. Thomas KC, Ellis AR, McLaurin C, Daniels J, Morrissey JP. Access to care for autism-related services. J Autism Dev Disord. 2007;37(10):1902-12.
105. Irvin DW, McBee M, Boyd BA, Hume K, Odom SL. Child and family factors associated with the use of services for preschoolers with autism spectrum disorder. Research in Autism Spectrum Disorders. 2012;6(1):565-72.

106. Zuckerman KE, Lindly OJ, Sinche BK, Nicolaidis C. Parent health beliefs, social determinants of health, and child health services utilization among U.S. school-age children with autism. Journal of developmental and behavioral pediatrics : JDBP. 2015;36(3):146-57.
107. Casagrande K, Ingersoll B. Service Delivery Outcomes in ASD: Role of Parent Education, Empowerment, and Professional Partnerships. Journal of Child & Family Studies. 2017;26(9):2386-95.
108. Durkin MS, Elsabbagh M, Barbaro J, Gladstone M, Happe F, Hoekstra RA, et al. Autism screening and diagnosis in low resource settings: Challenges and opportunities to enhance research and services worldwide. Autism research : official journal of the International Society for Autism Research. 2015;8(5):473-6.
109. Nathenson RA, Zablotsky B. The transition to the adult health care system among youths with Autism Spectrum Disorder. Psychiatric Services. 2017;68(7):735-8.
110. Mandell D, Ittenbach R, Levy S, Pinto-Martin J. Disparities in Diagnoses Received Prior to a Diagnosis of Autism Spectrum Disorder. Journal of Autism & Developmental Disorders. 2007;37(9):1795-802.
111. Zaroff CM, Uhm SY. Prevalence of autism spectrum disorders and influence of country of measurement and ethnicity. Social psychiatry and psychiatric epidemiology. 2012;47(3):395-8.
112. Magaña S, Parish SL, Rose RA, Timberlake M, Swaine JG. Racial and ethnic disparities in quality of health care among children with autism and other developmental disabilities. Intellectual and developmental disabilities. 2012;50(4):287-99.
113. Janz NK, Becker MH. The health belief model: A decade later. Health education quarterly. 1984;11(1):1-47.
114. Fishbein M, Ajzen I. Understanding attitudes and predicting social behavior. 1980.
115. Hewitt A, Hall-Lande J, Hamre K, Esler AN, Punyko J, Reichle J, et al. Autism Spectrum Disorder (ASD) Prevalence in Somali and Non-Somali Children. J Autism Dev Disord. 2016;46(8):2599-608.
116. Khanlou N, Haque N, Mustafa N, Vazquez LM, Mantini A, Weiss J. Access Barriers to Services by Immigrant Mothers of Children with Autism in Canada. International journal of mental health and addiction. 2017;15(2):239-59.
117. Al Anbar NN, Dardennes RM, Prado-Netto A, Kaye K, Contejean Y. Treatment choices in autism spectrum disorder: The role of parental illness perceptions. Research in developmental disabilities. 2010;31(3):817-28.
118. Chaidez V, Fernandez YGE, Wang LW, Angkustsiri K, Krakowiak P, Hertz-Picciotto I, et al. Comparison of maternal beliefs about causes of autism spectrum disorder and association with utilization of services and treatments. Child: care, health and development. 2018.
119. Gureje O, Lasebikan VO, Ephraim-Oluwanuga O, Olley BO, Kola L. Community study of knowledge of and attitude to mental illness in Nigeria. The British Journal of Psychiatry. 2005;186(5):436-41.
120. Bakare MO, Ebigbo PO, Agomoh AO, Eaton J, Onyeama GM, Okonkwo KO, et al. Knowledge about childhood autism and opinion among healthcare workers on availability of facilities and law caring for the needs and rights of children with childhood autism and other developmental disorders in Nigeria. BMC pediatrics. 2009;9(1):12.
121. Shyu Y-IL, Tsai J-L, Tsai W-C. Explaining and selecting treatments for autism: Parental explanatory models in Taiwan. Journal of autism and developmental disorders. 2010;40(11):1323-31.
122. Tilahun D, Hanlon C, Fekadu A, Tekola B, Baheretibeb Y, Hoekstra RA. Stigma, explanatory models and unmet needs of caregivers of children with developmental disorders in a low-income African country: a cross-sectional facility-based survey. BMC health services research. 2016;16:152.
123. Goin-Kochel RP, Mire SS, Dempsey AG. Emergence of autism spectrum disorder in children from simplex families: Relations to parental perceptions of etiology. Journal of autism and developmental disorders. 2015;45(5):1451-63.

124. Fischbach RL, Harris MJ, Ballan MS, Fischbach GD, Link BG. Is there concordance in attitudes and beliefs between parents and scientists about autism spectrum disorder? Autism : the international journal of research and practice. 2016;20(3):353-63.
125. Carlon S, Carter M, Stephenson J. A review of declared factors identified by parents of children with autism spectrum disorders (ASD) in making intervention decisions. Research in Autism Spectrum Disorders. 2013;7(2):369-81.
126. Gray DE. Perceptions of stigma: the parents of autistic children. Sociology of Health & Illness. 1993;15(1):102-20.
127. Broady TR, Stoyles GJ, Morse C. Understanding carers' lived experience of stigma: the voice of families with a child on the autism spectrum. Health & social care in the community. 2017;25(1):224-33.
128. Green S, Davis C, Karshmer E, Marsh P, Straight B. Living stigma: The impact of labeling, stereotyping, separation, status loss, and discrimination in the lives of individuals with disabilities and their families. Sociological Inquiry. 2005;75(2):197-215.
129. Fox F, Aabe N, Turner K, Redwood S, Rai D. "It was like walking without knowing where I was going": A Qualitative Study of Autism in a UK Somali Migrant Community. J Autism Dev Disord. 2017;47(2):305-15.
130. Ellen Selman L, Fox F, Aabe N, Turner K, Rai D, Redwood S. 'You are labelled by your children's disability' - A community-based, participatory study of stigma among Somali parents of children with autism living in the United Kingdom. Ethnicity & health. 2018;23(7):781-96.
131. Gona JK, Newton CR, Rimba K, Mapenzi R, Kihara M, Van de Vijver FJ, et al. Parents' and professionals' perceptions on causes and treatment options for Autism Spectrum Disorders (ASD) in a multicultural context on the Kenyan Coast. PloS one. 2015;10(8):e0132729.
132. Divan G, Vajaratkar V, Desai MU, Strik-Lievers L, Patel V. Challenges, Coping Strategies, and Unmet Needs of Families with a Child with Autism Spectrum Disorder in Goa, India. Autism Research. 2012;5(3):190-200.
133. Kiami SR, Goodgold S. Support Needs and Coping Strategies as Predictors of Stress Level among Mothers of Children with Autism Spectrum Disorder. Autism research and treatment. 2017;2017:8685950.
134. Schieve LA, Blumberg SJ, Rice C, Visser SN, Boyle C. The relationship between autism and parenting stress. Pediatrics. 2007;119(Supplement 1):S114-S21.
135. Bishop-Fitzpatrick L, Mazefsky CA, Minshew NJ, Eack SM. The relationship between stress and social functioning in adults with autism spectrum disorder and without intellectual disability. Autism Research. 2015;8(2):164-73.
136. Hoover DW. The effects of psychological trauma on children with autism spectrum disorders: a research review. Review Journal of Autism and Developmental Disorders. 2015;2(3):287-99.
137. Fung S, Lunsky Y, Weiss JA. Depression in youth with autism spectrum disorder: The role of ASD vulnerabilities and family–environmental stressors. Journal of Mental Health Research in Intellectual Disabilities. 2015;8(3-4):120-39.
138. Lunsky Y, Lin E, Balogh R, Klein-Geltink J, Wilton AS, Kurdyak P. Emergency department visits and use of outpatient physician services by adults with developmental disability and psychiatric disorder. Canadian journal of psychiatry Revue canadienne de psychiatrie. 2012;57(10):601-7.
139. Lunsky Y, Weiss JA, Paquette-Smith M, Durbin A, Tint A, Palucka AM, et al. Predictors of emergency department use by adolescents and adults with autism spectrum disorder: a prospective cohort study. BMJ open. 2017;7(7):e017377.
140. Matson JL, Nebel-Schwalm MS. Comorbid psychopathology with autism spectrum disorder in children: An overview. Research in developmental disabilities. 2007;28(4):341-52.

141. Buie T, Campbell DB, Fuchs GJ, Furuta GT, Levy J, VandeWater J, et al. Evaluation, diagnosis, and treatment of gastrointestinal disorders in individuals with ASDs: a consensus report. Pediatrics. 2010;125(Supplement 1):S1-S18.
142. Begeer S, El Bouk S, Boussaid W, Terwogt MM, Koot HM. Underdiagnosis and referral bias of autism in ethnic minorities. Journal of autism and developmental disorders. 2009;39(1):142.
143. Harrington JW, Rosen L, Garnecho A, Patrick PA. Parental perceptions and use of complementary and alternative medicine practices for children with autistic spectrum disorders in private practice. Journal of Developmental & Behavioral Pediatrics. 2006;27(2):S156-S61.
144. Hanson E, Kalish LA, Bunce E, Curtis C, McDaniel S, Ware J, et al. Use of complementary and alternative medicine among children diagnosed with autism spectrum disorder. Journal of autism and developmental disorders. 2007;37(4):628-36.
145. Perrin JM, Coury DL, Hyman SL, Cole L, Reynolds AM, Clemons T. Complementary and alternative medicine use in a large pediatric autism sample. Pediatrics. 2012;130(Supplement 2):S77-S82.
146. Wong HH, Smith RG. Patterns of complementary and alternative medical therapy use in children diagnosed with autism spectrum disorders. Journal of autism and developmental disorders. 2006;36(7):901-9.
147. Bowker A, D'Angelo NM, Hicks R, Wells K. Treatments for autism: Parental choices and perceptions of change. Journal of Autism and Developmental Disorders. 2011;41(10):1373-82.
148. Akins CRS, Krakowiak P, Angkustsiri K, Hertz-Picciotto I, Hansen RL. Utilization patterns of conventional and complementary/alternative treatments in children with autism spectrum disorders and developmental disabilities in a population-based study. Journal of developmental and behavioral pediatrics: JDBP. 2014;35(1):1.
149. Kogan MD, Strickland BB, Blumberg SJ, Singh GK, Perrin JM, van Dyck PC. A national profile of the health care experiences and family impact of autism spectrum disorder among children in the United States, 2005–2006. Pediatrics. 2008;122(6):e1149-e58.
150. Vohra R, Madhavan S, Sambamoorthi U, St Peter C. Access to services, quality of care, and family impact for children with autism, other developmental disabilities, and other mental health conditions. Autism : the international journal of research and practice. 2014;18(7):815-26.
151. Summers JA, Hoffman L, Marquis J, Turnbull A, Poston D. Relationship between parent satisfaction regarding partnerships with professionals and age of child. Topics in Early Childhood Special Education. 2005;25(1):48-58.
152. Burkett K, Morris E, Manning-Courtney P, Anthony J, Shambley-Ebron D. African American Families on Autism Diagnosis and Treatment: The Influence of Culture. Journal of Autism & Developmental Disorders. 2015;45(10):3244-54.
153. Detmar SB, Muller MJ, Schornagel JH, Wever LD, Aaronson NK. Health-related quality-of-life assessments and patient-physician communication: a randomized controlled trial. Jama. 2002;288(23):3027-34.
154. Parish S, Magana S, Rose R, Timberlake M, Swaine JG. Health care of Latino children with autism and other developmental disabilities: quality of provider interaction mediates utilization. American journal on intellectual and developmental disabilities. 2012;117(4):304-15.
155. Bakare MO, Agomoh AO, Ebigbo PO, Eaton J, Okonkwo KO, Onwukwe JU, et al. Etiological explanation, treatability and preventability of childhood autism: a survey of Nigerian healthcare workers' opinion. Annals of General Psychiatry. 2009;8(1):6.
156. Broadbent E, Petrie KJ, Main J, Weinman J. The brief illness perception questionnaire. Journal of psychosomatic research. 2006;60(6):631-7.
157. Weiss JA, Lunsky Y. The Brief Family Distress Scale: A Measure of Crisis in Caregivers of Individuals with Autism Spectrum Disorders. Journal of Child and Family Studies. 2011;20(4):521-8.

158. Mantopoulos J, Webster TR, Bradley EH, Jackson E, Cole-Lewis H, Kidane L, et al. A brief questionnaire for assessing patient healthcare experiences in low-income settings. International Journal for Quality in Health Care. 2011;23(3):258-68.
159. Marshall GN, Hays RD. The patient satisfaction questionnaire short-form (PSQ-18). Rand Santa Monica, CA; 1994.
160. Mire SS, Tolar TD, Brewton CM, Raff NS, McKee SL. Validating the revised illness perception questionnaire as a measure of parent perceptions of autism spectrum disorder. Journal of autism and developmental disorders. 2018;48(5):1761-79.
161. Thayaparan AJ, Mahdi EJ. The Patient Satisfaction Questionnaire Short Form (PSQ-18) as an adaptable, reliable, and validated tool for use in various settings. Medical education online. 2013;18.
162. Webster TR, Mantopoulos J, Jackson E, Cole-Lewis H, Kidane L, Kebede S, et al. A brief questionnaire for assessing patient healthcare experiences in low-income settings. International Journal for Quality in Health Care. 2011;23(3):258-68.
163. AAP Developmental and Behavioral Pediatrics. Voigt RG, Macias MM, Myers SM, editors2010. 612 p.
164. Bakare MO, Munir KM. Autism spectrum disorders (ASD) in Africa: a perspective. African journal of psychiatry. 2011;14(3):208-10.
165. Sawni A. Attention-deficit/hyperactivity disorder and complementary/alternative medicine. Adolescent medicine: state of the art reviews. 2008;19(2):313-26, xi.
166. Bethell CD, Kogan MD, Strickland BB, Schor EL, Robertson J, Newacheck PW. A national and state profile of leading health problems and health care quality for US children: key insurance disparities and across-state variations. Academic pediatrics. 2011;11(3):S22-S33.
167. Mandell DS, Wiggins LD, Carpenter LA, Daniels J, DiGuiseppi C, Durkin MS, et al. Racial/Ethnic Disparities in the Identification of Children With Autism Spectrum Disorders. American Journal of Public Health. 2009;99(3):493-8.
168. Meyers MK, Lukemeyer A, Smeeding T. The cost of caring: Childhood disability and poor families. Social Service Review. 1998;72(2):209-33.
169. Birenbaum A, Guyot D, Cohen HJ. Health care financing for severe developmental disabilities. Monographs of the American Association on Mental Retardation. 1990(14):1.

## APPENDIX 1
## QUESTIONNAIRE ON HEALTH SERVICE USE IN CHILDREN WITH ASD/GDD

Date: ______________________________

Telephone contact ___________________

### 1.0 SOCIODEMOGRAPHIC AND ECONOMIC CHARACTERISTICS

*Please respond the statements in the table below regarding your family by ticking where appropriate.*

| Code | 1 | 2 | 3 | 4 | 5 | 6 |
|---|---|---|---|---|---|---|
| Who is the primary caregiver for child? | Biologic mother | Foster mother | Aunt | Grand mother | Father | Other |
| Primary caregiver's age group (years) | < 25 | 25 – 30 | 31 - 35 | 36 - 40 | 41- 45 | >45 |
| Marital status of caregiver | Married | Living with a partner | Single | Separated | Divorced | |
| Nationality of caregiver | South Africa | Congo | Botswana | Malawi | Zimbabwe | other |
| Ancestry of caregiver | White | Black | Coloured/ mixed | Indian | other | |
| Language spoken at home | English | Afrikaans | Xhosa | Mixed | Other | |
| Type of neighbourhood you reside at? | Low income (Shack, windy house) | Middle income (Rentals, stone wall) | High income (stone wall, flats) | | | |
| How many children (<6yrs old), live in your household | 1 | 2 | 3 | 4 | 5 | 6 |
| Where does child spend most of their day? | At home | Day-care | Friend's place | relative's place | Neighbour's | Creche |
| Mean family income per month (Rands) | <2000 | 2000-3999 | 4000 - 5999 | 6000 -7999 | 8000 - 9999 | >10,000 |
| Is mum in employment or studying? | Un-employed | Self-employed | Informal - jobs | Formal – part-time job | Formal- full time job | Studying |
| Is dad in employment or away from home? | Un-employed | Self-employed | Informal-employment | Formal – part-time | Formal- full time | Studying |
| Does you receive any child support grant? | None | Social security support grant | Care dependency grant | Other | | |
| Highest level of education attained by carer? | None | Primary | Secondary | Tertiary college | University | |

| How long does it take you to come to Red cross Hospital (hrs) | 1 | 2 | 3 | 4 | 5 | 6 |
|---|---|---|---|---|---|---|
| How much does it cost you to come to Red Cross Hosp and back home (Rands) | None | < 50 | 50- 99 | 100 -149 | 150 -200 | >200 |
| What means of transport do you use to bring child to hospital? | Walk | Public transport | Own car | Taxi-private | Train | Other |
| Do you have a helper that can bring child to hospital if you are unable to? | No | Sometimes | Always have someone to assist | | | |
| How do you pay for child's healthcare? | State paid | Medical aid | Private insurance | Family | Other | |
| Did child spend the last 1yr in Western Cape province? | Yes, here all through | Away for <2 weeks | Away for 2- 4 weeks | Away for 5-8 weeks | Away for 9-12 weeks | Away for >16 weeks |

### 1.1 CHILD CHARACTERISTICS

*Please provide us information about the child in table below.*

| Code | 1 | 2 | 3 | 4 | 5 | 6 |
|---|---|---|---|---|---|---|
| Birth order | 1st born | 2nd born | 3rd born | 4th born | 5th born | Other |
| Child's age (years) | 2 < 3 | 3 < 4 | 4 < 5 | 5 < 6 | 6 < 7 | |
| Gender | Male | Female | | | | |
| Core diagnosis | Autism (ASD) | Global dev delay (GDD) | ASD/ ADHD | ASD/ GDD | GDD/ ADHD | |
| Level of severity | Level 1/ Mild | Level 2/ Moderate | Level 3/ Severe | | | |
| Age at first diagnosis | <1yr | 1≤ 2yr | 2 ≤ 3yr | 3 ≤ 4yr | 4 ≤ 5yr | >5 |
| Where was diagnosis was first made | Red Cross Hosp | Day Hosp | Baby Clinic | Private doctor | Therapist | |
| Time taken from parent concern to diagnosis | 1 ≤ 2yr | 2 ≤ 3yr | 3 ≤ 4yr | 4 ≤ 5yr | 5 ≤ 6yr | |
| Does child have any chronic medical problems? | None | Asthma | HIV | Tuberculosis | Seizures | Other |
| Does child have any underlying condition(s) | None | Genetic syndrome | Metabolic | Hormonal | Structural defects | Other |
| Has child received all primary immunizations | Up to date | Missed >1 vaccine (s) | None | Unclear | | |
| How's the child's speech? | Non-verbal (No spoken words) | Few words (< 10) with meaning | 10 ≤ 20 words, No phrases | 20–30 words, 2- 3 word phrases | > 30 words, Sentences with errors | Fluent speech |

## 2.0 HEALTH SERVICE USAGE PATTERNS

2.1 Did you attend any therapy for the condition last year?
1. Yes [ ] 2. No [ ] 3.Cannot remember [ ]

2.2 If yes, where does child attend these services?
RXH [ ] 2. Day hospital [ ] 3. Private [ ] 4. Other ]____________________

*(For questions 2.3 -2.8 please indicate your response in table below)*

2.3 Did you get any appointments for therapy or other support services in the last 1 month, and how many times did you attend in last 1 month and then in last 1year?

2.4 Did you need a service but could not access it or missed the appointment in last 1 year?

| | | Number of clinics attended | | Unmet service needs in past 1 year | |
|---|---|---|---|---|---|
| | | Last 1 month | Past 1 year | Needed but not accessed | Missed appoint ments |
| | **Core therapies** | | | | |
| 1 | Speech/language therapist | | | | |
| 2 | Occupational therapist | | | | |
| 3 | Physiotherapist | | | | |
| | *Sub- total core visits* | | | | |
| | **Auxiliary services** | | | | |
| 4 | Audiology | | | | |
| 5 | Social worker | | | | |
| 6 | Family counsellor | | | | |
| 7 | Pharmacy | | | | |
| 8 | EEG | | | | |
| | *Sub- total ancillary visits* | | | | |

2.5 Please indicate main reason(s) for missing any booked sessions in the last year.
*[speech therapy (SLT), occupational therapy (OT), physiotherapy (PT), audiology (AD), Social worker (SW), family counsellor (FC), pharmacy (PH)}*

| | **Reasons for missed sessions** | **Core therapy sessions** | | | **Ancillary services** | | | |
|---|---|---|---|---|---|---|---|---|
| | | **SLT** | **OT** | **PT** | **AD** | **SW** | **FC** | **Ph** |
| | | 1 | 2 | 3 | 4 | 5 | 6 | 7 |
| 1 | None missed | | | | | | | |
| 2 | Forgot appointment date | | | | | | | |
| 3 | Appointment date not communicated on time. | | | | | | | |
| 4 | Was late for appointment | | | | | | | |
| 5 | Had to attend work or other duties | | | | | | | |
| 6 | Did not have transport/fare to go | | | | | | | |
| 7 | Did not have any social support | | | | | | | |
| 8 | Child was unwell | | | | | | | |
| 9 | Bad whether | | | | | | | |
| 10 | Travelled out of Cape Town | | | | | | | |
| 11 | Other | | | | | | | |

**EMERGENCY SERVICES (medical and mental health problems)**

2.6 Did this child experience any emergency medical problems/injuries or behavioural problems last 1 year?
1. No [ ] 2. Yes [ ] 3. Cannot remember [ ]

2.7 Please indicate in the table below the emergency problem(s) that brought child to hospital, number of visits and facility visited in last 1 year.
*(ED RXH= Emergency dept RXH, Dev clinic RXH = Development clinic at RXH, CDH= Community day Hospital)*

| | | | **Where service was sought** | | | | |
|---|---|---|---|---|---|---|---|
| | Code | Number of visits last 1 year | ED - RXH | Dev clinic - RXH | CDH | Private facility | Chemist |
| | | | 1 | 2 | 3 | 4 | 5 |
| **Medical conditions** | | | | | | | |
| None | 0 | | | | | | |
| Vomiting, diarrhoea, constipation, poor feeding. | 1 | | | | | | |
| Seizures/epilepsy | 2 | | | | | | |
| Sleeping problems | 3 | | | | | | |
| Allergies | 4 | | | | | | |
| Infection/fever | 5 | | | | | | |
| Cough/flu/Pneumonia | 6 | | | | | | |
| Trauma/Accidents (falls, bruises, cuts, burns) | 7 | | | | | | |
| To collect medications | 8 | | | | | | |
| *Total medical visits* | | | | | | | |
| **Mental health problems** | | | | | | | |
| None | 0 | | | | | | |
| Hyperactive, distracted, impulsive | 1 | | | | | | |
| Overly anxious | 2 | | | | | | |
| Overly excited | 3 | | | | | | |
| Mood swings | 4 | | | | | | |
| Withdrawn, not talking or feeding | 5 | | | | | | |
| Aggression | 6 | | | | | | |
| Irritability or agitation | 7 | | | | | | |
| Very rigid behaviours | 8 | | | | | | |
| Very restricted behaviours | 9 | | | | | | |
| Elopement/escape/ wandering off | 10 | | | | | | |
| Self-injurious behaviours | 11 | | | | | | |
| *Total behaviour visits* | | | | | | | |
| ***Total emergencies*** | | | | | | | |

2.8 Did child ever require emergency services, but you could not access on it time?
1. No [ ] 2. Yes [ ] 3. I don't remember [ ]

2.9 Please indicate what time of day you sought emergency services for the child and for what condition and whether the child required an overnight stay or admission?

| | | Timing of emergency services | | | Hospital stay | |
|---|---|---|---|---|---|---|
| | | Working hrs (8am - 5 pm) | Late hours (6pm- 8am) | Week- ends (anytime) | Over-night stay (<12hrs) | Admission for >24 hrs |
| | | 1 | 2 | 3 | 1 | 2 |
| **Medical conditions** | | | | | | |
| None | 0 | | | | | |
| Vomiting, diarrhoea, constipation, poor feeding. | 1 | | | | | |
| Seizures/fits | 2 | | | | | |
| Sleeping problems | 3 | | | | | |
| Allergies | 4 | | | | | |
| Child infections /fever | 5 | | | | | |
| Cough/flu/Pneumonia | 6 | | | | | |
| Trauma/Accidents (falls, bruises, cuts, burns) | 7 | | | | | |
| To collect medications | 8 | | | | | |
| *Total medical visits* | | | | | | |
| **Mental health problems** | 9 | | | | | |
| *Total behaviour visits* | | | | | | |

**MEDICAL SPECIALIST CLINICS**

2.10 Please indicate in table below how many times you got specialists' appointments, and number of specialist clinics attended in last 1 year?
2.11 Did you need any specialist services, but did not receive it for whatever reason?

| | | Specialist clinics | | Unmet specialist needs | |
|---|---|---|---|---|---|
| **Specialist clinics** | | Booked clinics | Clinics attended | Needed but not accessed | Missed booked appointment |
| None | 0 | | | | |
| Development | 1 | | | | |
| Neurology | 2 | | | | |
| Psychiatry | 3 | | | | |
| Genetics | 4 | | | | |
| Ophthalmologist | 5 | | | | |
| Gastroenterology | 6 | | | | |
| Pulmonology | 7 | | | | |
| Allergy | 8 | | | | |
| Cardiology | 9 | | | | |
| Ear-Nose-throat clinic | 10 | | | | |
| Surgeons | 11 | | | | |
| Others (Specify) | 12 | | | | |
| Total visits | | | | | |

**WELL BABY CLINICS**

2.12 Did the child ever attend any well baby services?
Please indicate in table how many times you ever went to hospital for primary care services listed in the table below.

| | | Number of times |
|---|---|---|
| Code | None | |
| 0 | Growth monitoring/ development screening only | |
| 1 | Flu vaccine | |
| 2 | Other vaccinations | |
| 3 | Health advice/education | |
| 4 | Other concerns | |
| 5 | | |

## 3.0 DRUGS AND COMPLEMENTARY THERAPY USE

3.1 Has child been on any medications used regularly in the past year?
Please indicate which ones you have used in the table below?

| | **Psychotropics drugs** | **Yes** | | **Other conventional drugs** | **Yes** |
|---|---|---|---|---|---|
| 0 | None | | 0 | None | |
| 1 | Risperidone | | 1 | Inhalers (MDIs) | |
| 2 | Methylphenidate | | 2 | Skin topicals | |
| 3 | Valproate (Epilim) | | 3 | Laxatives | |
| 4 | Phenobarbitone | | 4 | Anti - tuberculosis | |
| 5 | Carbamazepine | | 5 | Omeprazole | |
| 6 | Other antiepileptic drugs | | 6 | Prednisolone | |
| 7 | Antidepressants | | 7 | HIV meds | |
| 8 | Antipsychotics | | 8 | Immune modifiers | |
| 9 | Melatonin | | 9 | Hormones | |
| 10 | Other | | 10 | Others (Specify) | |

3.2 Did you use any supplements, diets, or therapies other than those prescribed in hospital in past year? Please indicate which ones and how often they were used in table below?

| | CAM use | Code | Yes | Occasional (1) | Often (2) | Always (3) |
|---|---|---|---|---|---|---|
| Diet therapy | None | 0 | | | | |
| | Dairy restrictions | 1 | | | | |
| | Casein free diets | 2 | | | | |
| | No sugar diets | 3 | | | | |
| | Omega 3 supplements | 4 | | | | |
| | Magnesium supplements | 5 | | | | |
| | Vitamin supplements | 6 | | | | |
| | Other diets (Specify) | 7 | | | | |
| Other therapies | Spiritual healing | 1 | | | | |
| | Acupuncture | 2 | | | | |
| | Zomotherapy | 3 | | | | |
| | Yoga | 4 | | | | |
| | Traditional healers | 5 | | | | |
| | Hippotherapy | 6 | | | | |
| | Cannabis | 7 | | | | |
| Others | | 8 | | | | |

### 4.1 CAREGIVER PERSPECTIVES

*On a scale of 0 to 4, with 0 being the lowest score and 4 the highest,*
*please indicate what you feel about the child's illness by ticking in the table below.*

| | **Brief illness perception questionnaire** | 0 | 1 | 2 | 3 | 4 |
|---|---|---|---|---|---|---|
| | | | | | | |
| 1 | How much does the illness affect your life? | | | | | |
| 2 | How long do you think the illness will continue? | | | | | |
| 3 | How much control do you feel you have over the illness? | | | | | |
| 4 | How much do you think the treatments can help the child's illness | | | | | |
| 5 | How severe are the symptoms in the child? | | | | | |
| 6 | How concerned are you about the illness? | | | | | |
| 7 | How well do you understand the illness? | | | | | |
| 8 | How much does the illness affect you emotionally? (Does it make you angry, scared, upset, anxious, depressed?) | | | | | |
| 9 | Please list in rank-order the 3 most important factors that you believe caused the illness | | | | | |
| | 1. | | | | | |
| | 2. | | | | | |
| | 3. | | | | | |

### 4.2 FAMILY STRESS LEVEL

*Caring for a child with special needs can be demanding and stressful on the family.*
*Please rate where you and your family currently are in terms of coping by ticking in the appropriate box in table below?*

| Code | Family distress score | **Tick** |
|---|---|---|
| 1 | Everything is fine. Not in a crisis at all | |
| 2 | Everything is fine, but sometimes we have difficulties | |
| 3 | Things are sometimes stressful, but we can deal with problems if they arise | |
| 4 | Things are very stressful, but we are managing to deal with the problems when they arise | |
| 5 | Things are very stressful, but we are getting by with a lot of effort. | |
| 6 | We have to work extremely hard every moment of everyday to avoid having a crisis | |
| 7 | We won't be able to handle things soon. If one more thing goes wrong, we will be in a crisis | |
| 8 | We are currently in a crisis, but we are dealing with it ourselves | |
| 9 | We are currently in a crisis, and have asked for help from crisis services | |
| 10 | We are currently in a crisis and it could not get any worse | |
| | | |

**4.3 EXPERIENCES IN HEALTH SERVICES**

Please rate your experiences in various service areas at Red Cross hospital (RXH) or Community day hospitals (CDH) in the table below.

*(Use scale of 0 - 4, where 0 = Not satisfied, 1= somewhat dissatisfied, 2= somewhat satisfied, 3= satisfied, 4= very satisfied)*

| | | Therapy services | | Support services, RXH | Specialist clinics, RXH |
|---|---|---|---|---|---|
| | | RXH | CDH | | |
| | ***Communication with nurses/provider*** | | | | |
| 1 | Treat patients with courtesy and respect | | | | |
| 2 | Listened carefully | | | | |
| 3 | Explain things in an understandable way | | | | |
| 4 | Understand child's behaviour, are empathetic | | | | |
| 5 | Are efficient | | | | |
| | ***Communication with doctors*** | | | | |
| 6 | Treat patients with courtesy and respect | | | | |
| 7 | Listen carefully | | | | |
| 8 | Explain things in an understandable way | | | | |
| 9 | Understand child's behaviour, are empathetic | | | | |
| 10 | Are efficient | | | | |
| | ***Physical environment*** | | | | |
| 11 | Therapy room is kept clean and in order | | | | |
| 12 | Surrounding area/toilet are clean | | | | |
| | ***Management of disruptive behaviour*** | | | | |
| **13** | Staff did everything they could to help | | | | |
| **14** | Provided a safe environment for child | | | | |
| | ***Medication/therapy communication*** | | | | |
| 15 | Clearly explained each intervention given | | | | |
| 16 | Explained possible drug side effects | | | | |
| | **Please rate the overall quality services** | | | | |

## 4.4 LEVEL OF SATISFACTION

*Please read each of the statements carefully and tell us your feelings about the care you are receiving currently, whether good or bad.*

*By rating on a scale of 0-4, how strongly do you agree or disagree with the following statements by marking in the table below?*

1. *Strongly disagree*
2. *Disagree*
3. *Uncertain*
4. *Agree*
5. *Strongly agree*

| | | 1 | 2 | 3 | 4 | 5 |
|---|---|---|---|---|---|---|
| 1 | Doctors are good about explaining reasons for medical tests | | | | | |
| 2 | Doctor's office had everything I needed to provide diagnosis | | | | | |
| 3 | The medical care I have been receiving is just about perfect | | | | | |
| 4 | Sometimes doctors make me wonder if their diagnosis is correct | | | | | |
| 5 | I feel confident that I can get the medical care I need without being set back financially | | | | | |
| 6 | When I go for medical care, they are careful to check everything when treating or examining me | | | | | |
| 7 | I have to pay for more of my medical care than I can afford | | | | | |
| 8 | I have easy access to medical specialists I need | | | | | |
| 9 | Where I get care, people have to wait too long for emergency treatment | | | | | |
| 10 | Doctors act too business-like and impersonal to me | | | | | |
| 11 | Doctors treat me in a friendly and courteous manner | | | | | |
| 12 | Those who provide my medical care sometimes hurry too much when they treat me | | | | | |
| 13 | Doctors sometimes ignore what I tell them | | | | | |
| 14 | I have some doubts about the ability of the doctors to treat me | | | | | |
| 15 | Doctors usually spent plenty of time with me | | | | | |
| 16 | I find it hard to get appointment for medical care right away | | | | | |
| 17 | I am dissatisfied with some things about the care I receive | | | | | |
| 18 | Am able to get medical care whenever I need it | | | | | |
| | Others | | | | | |

**APPENDIX 2**

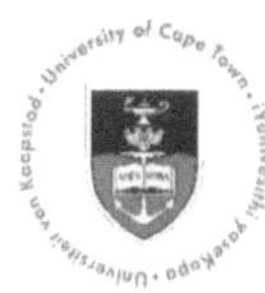


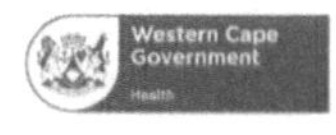


## DEPARTMENT OF PAEDIATRICS AND CHILD HEALTH

---

Division of Developmental Paediatrics
University of Cape Town
Red Cross War Memorial Children's Hospital
Klipfontein Road
Rondebosch
7700

## CONSENT FORM FOR HEALTH SERVICE UTILIZATION PROJECT

***PRINCIPLE INVESTIGATOR:*** *Dr. Florence Oringe*
***ADDRESS:*** *School of Child and Adolescent Health, Red Cross Children's Hospital, and the University of Cape Town*
***INVESTIGATORS CONTACTS:*** *0769501139*
***TITLE:*** *Health service utilization patterns by pre-school children with autism spectrum disorder in South Africa, a comparison with global developmental delay*

Dear participant,
Research has shown that children with developmental disorders have very complex health care needs and there are significant disparities in health services access in these children worldwide. We are undertaking a research study whose aim is to better understand how existing health services are utilized by children with autism or global developmental delays, in order to identify any gaps in care, to assess level of satisfaction of clients and to identify access challenges. The findings will inform improvement of service delivery for these children. We invite your participation in the study. Participation is voluntary and there are no consequences of declining to participate.

**Why have you been invited to participate?**
Your child is one of those accessing services at Red Cross Children's Hospital for the developmental conditions under investigation. As one of our clients, your participation is highly appreciated.

**What are the procedures to be followed?**
The researcher will access the child's medical records to establish the diagnosis. You will subsequently be engaged in a 30- 45-minute interview where you will be requested

to respond to questions regarding your household and child characteristics, your patterns of attendance to various departments for the child, your experiences and levels of family coping and any access challenges and then report on your level of satisfaction with our services in the past one year.

**Who will have access to your child's medical records?**

Only members of the research team will have access to the child's records and hospital attendance data. All information will remain confidential and if the results of this study are published individual participants will not be identified.

**Are there any risks involved in your child taking part in this research?**

No. There is no harm that will be caused to the child or yourself. Some questions asked during the interview may be personal, regarding access challenges and stress levels at home. However, you are free not answer or to discontinue the interview at any time.

**Will the child benefit from taking part in this research?**

Participation in this study has no financial or personal benefits. However, the information obtained will be used to improve health service provision for these children in future.

**What protection is in place for the research participant opinions**

Your identity by name will not be used on the research questionnaires. Instead you will be identified by study numbers to maintain confidentiality. No one will be victimized for their opinion.

**Will this benefit children from our own community?**

Yes. Findings will inform service delivery for children with similar conditions seeking health services in public services in Western Cape province.

**How will my privacy and confidentiality be guaranteed?**

Interviews will be conducted in a private consultation room. Utmost confidentiality will always be maintained, and information shared will only be used for purposes of this study and for publication of the research findings.

If you have any questions you may contact the principle investigator Dr. Oringe whose contacts are provided above or Prof. Kirsty, Head of Department of developmental Pediatrics, Red Cross Hospital and UCT.

**Respondent's statement**

I have understood the information above and the terms of my participation in this study: I have been given a chance to ask questions for clarification which has been answered satisfactorily. I voluntarily choose to participate in this study. I understand that the information I will provide will be treated with confidentiality and kept private. I understand I can refuse to proceed with the interview at any time without any consequences.

Signing or thumb printing.

Date ____________________

**Interviewer's statement**

I, the undersigned have explained to the respondent the procedures in the study, the benefits and the risks involved in participating in the study in a language she understands.

Name of interviewer ____________________________________

Interviewer signature ____________________ Date __________________

## APPENDIX 3

### Supplemental information

**Correlation of other factors with health care utilization (a) overall; (b) restricted to children with primary diagnosis of ASD; and (c) restricted to children with primary diagnosis of GDD: mean differences with 95%CI from linear regression**

| | (a) Full cohort (N=240) | | (b) Children with GDD (n=124) | | (c) Children with ASD (n=116) | |
|---|---|---|---|---|---|---|
| | Crude *β* coefficient (95% CI) | *p* | Crude *β* coefficient (95% CI) | *p* | Crude *β* coefficient (95% CI) | *p* |
| Nationality | | | | | | |
| *Non-South African (ref)* | 1.00 | - | 1.00 | - | 1.00 | - |
| *South African* | -0.04 (-2.03; 1.96) | 0.97 | -0.38 (-3.65; 2.89) | 0.82 | -0.23 (-2.68; 2.22) | 0.85 |
| Chronic comorbid diagnosis | | | | | | |
| *No other known chronic diagnosis* | 1.00 | - | 1.00 | - | 1.00 | - |
| *≥1 other chronic diagnosis* | 0.95 (-0.68; 2.58) | 0.25 | 0.98 (-1.18; 3.14) | 0.37 | -1.23 (-4.22; 1.76) | 0.42 |
| Speech development | | | | | | |
| *Speaks >20 words and phrases* | 1.00 | - | 1.00 | - | 1.00 | - |
| *Non-verbal, ≤ 20 or no phrases* | -0.67 (-2.38; 1.05) | 0.44 | 0.35 (-1.94; 2.65) | 0.76 | -1.40 (-4.15; 1.35) | 0.31 |
| ***Brief illness perspective questionnaire (B-IPQ)*** | | | | | | |
| Consequences | -0.52 (-1.41; 0.38) | 0.26 | -0.43 (-1.61; 0.75) | 0.47 | -0.42 (-1.83; 0.99) | 0.56 |
| Timeline | -0.35 (-1.29; 0.59) | 0.46 | -0.15 (-1.40; 1.09) | 0.81 | -0.41 (-1.87; 1.06) | 0.58 |
| Personal control | 0.53 (-0.16; 1.23) | 0.13 | -0.27 (-1.35; 0.81) | 0.62 | 1.18 (0.30-2.05) | 0.009 |
| Treatment control | 1.07 (0.38; 1.76) | 0.003 | 0.14 (-0.94; 1.22) | 0.79 | 1.79 (0.94; 2.64) | <0.0001 |
| Identity | 0.67 (-0.16; 1.50) | 0.11 | 0.56 (-0.68; 1.81) | 0.37 | 0.73 (-0.36; 1.82) | 0.19 |
| Understanding | 0.32 (-0.33; 0.96) | 0.33 | -0.23 (-1.18; 0.72) | 0.63 | 0.78 (-0.08; 1.64) | 0.08 |
| Emotional response | -0.50 (-1.19; 0.20) | 0.16 | -0.08 (-1.07; 0.92) | 0.88 | -0.88 (-1.83; 0.08) | 0.07 |

| | | | | | | |
|---|---|---|---|---|---|---|
| ***Experiences in Health Services*** | | | | | | |
| Communication with therapist | 0.38 (-1.03; 1.79) | 0.60 | 0.92 (-1.12; 2.96) | 0.37 | 0.21 (-1.64; 2.06) | 0.82 |
| Communication with doctor | 0.61 (-0.84; 2.06) | 0.41 | 0.67 (-1.40; 2.75) | 0.52 | 0.54 (-1.43; 2.51) | 0.59 |
| Physical environment | 0.72 (-0.52; 1.96) | 0.26 | 1.26 (-0.49; 3.01) | 0.16 | 0.43 (-1.17; 2.04) | 0.59 |
| Management of disruptive behaviour | -0.04 (-1.22; 1.14) | 0.95 | 0.87 (-0.86; 2.60) | 0.32 | -0.56 (-2.02; 0.90) | 0.45 |
| Therapy communication | 0.16 (-0.96; 1.27) | 0.78 | 0.77 (-0.87; 2.41) | 0.35 | -0.25 (-1.64; 1.14) | 0.72 |
| ***Patient satisfaction questionnaire (PSQ-18)*** | | | | | | |
| General satisfaction | 0.36 (-0.82; 1.55) | 0.55 | -0.64 (-2.11; 0.82) | 0.38 | 1.45 (-0.09; 2.99) | 0.06 |
| Technical quality | 0.52 (-0.63; 1.67) | 0.38 | 0.08 (-1.49; 1.66) | 0.92 | 0.29 (-1.25 1.83) | 0.71 |
| Interpersonal manner | 0.08 (-1.04; 1.20) | 0.89 | -0.76 (-2.31; 0.80) | 0.34 | 0.18 (-1.25; 1.60) | 0.81 |
| Communication | 0.82 (-0.37; 2.01) | 0.18 | 0.47 (-1.29; 2.24) | 0.60 | 1.31 (-0.24; 2.86) | 0.10 |
| Financial status | 0.07 (-0.94; 1.07) | 0.90 | 0.21 (-1.25; 1.67) | 0.78 | 0.17 (-1.12; 1.46) | 0.80 |
| Time spent with doctor | 0.66 (-0.42; 1.74) | 0.23 | 0.34 (-1.09; 1.78) | 0.64 | 0.45 (-1.04; 1.94) | 0.55 |
| Accessibility and convenience | 0.25 (-0.68; 1.19) | 0.59 | -0.34 (-1.57; 0.89) | 0.59 | 0.77 (-0.48; 2.02) | 0.22 |
| Satisfaction overall | 0.12 (-0.13; 0.37) | 0.35 | -0.06 (-0.42; 0.30) | 0.74 | 0.29 (-0.04; 0.62) | 0.09 |

Abbreviations: GDD, global developmental disorder; ASD, autism spectrum disorder; CI, confidence interval, Beta-coefficients represent mean difference in health care visits: comparing each category to the reference, or difference per unit increase for continuous variables

[1] *p*-value for interaction effect of indicated variable (e.g. child sex) with binary indicator for primary diagnosis (GDD vs ASD) is $p<0.05$, indicating likely presence of effect measure modification, i.e. $p<0.05$ suggests that the relationship between indicated variable and overall health care visits varies within subgroups of primary diagnosis

www.ingramcontent.com/pod-product-compliance
Lightning Source LLC
LaVergne TN
LVHW041458190726
843491LV00008B/2429

* 9 7 8 3 3 8 4 2 5 4 3 7 5 *